THE EASY SUGAR DETOX COOKBOOK

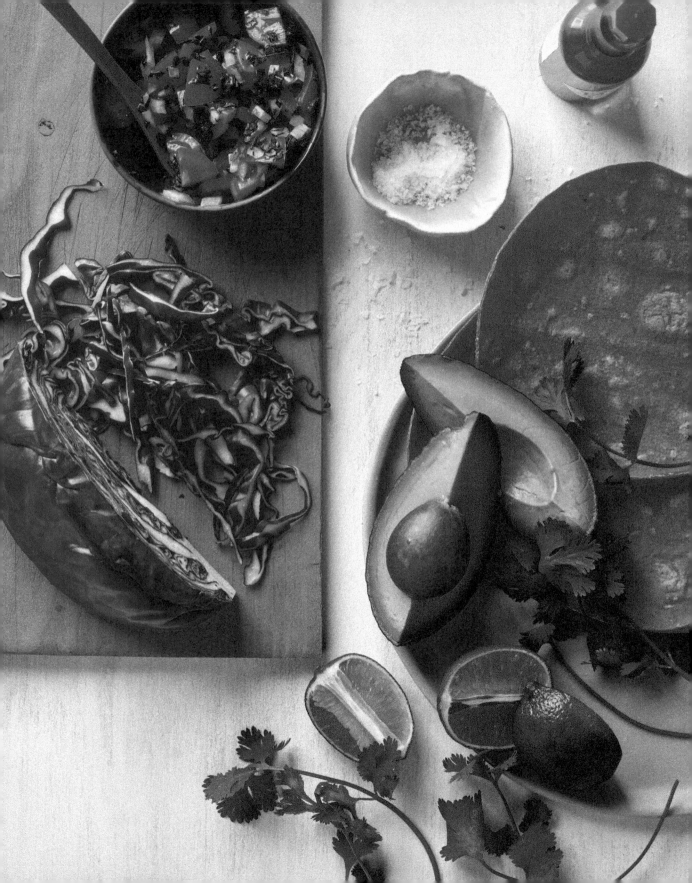

THE EASY
Sugar Detox
COOKBOOK

125 RECIPES
FOR A SUGAR-FREE LIFESTYLE

KRISTEN YARKER, MSc, RD

PHOTOGRAPHY BY ANNABELLE BREAKEY

ROCKRIDGE PRESS

For general information on our other products and services or to obtain techni-cal support, please contact our Customer Care Department within the U.S. at (866) 744-2665, or outside the U.S. at (510) 253-0500.

Rockridge Press publishes its books in a variety of electronic and print formats. Some content that appears in print may not be available in electronic books, and vice versa.

Interior and Cover Designer: Diana Haas
Art Producer: Michael Hardgrove
Editor: Daniel Grogan
Production Editor: Andrew Yackira
Production Manager: Giraud Lorber
Photography: Annabelle Breakey
Food Styling: Abby Stolfo

ISBN: Print 978-1-64152-787-3 | eBook 978-1-64152-788-0
R0

To Grannie. For sitting with me
on the back steps, shucking corn and
snapping green beans. Teaching me
that cooking equals love.

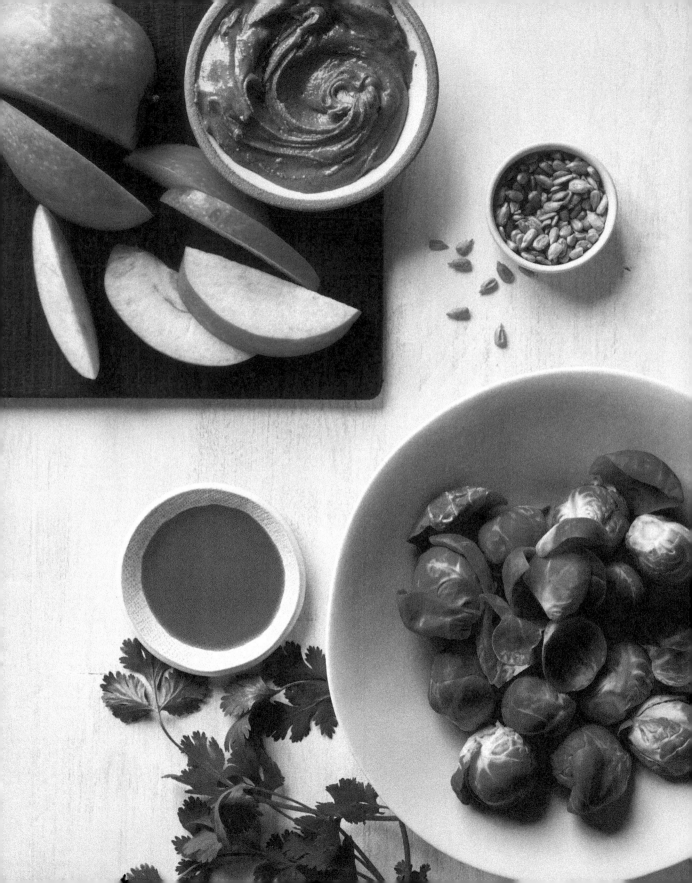

CONTENTS

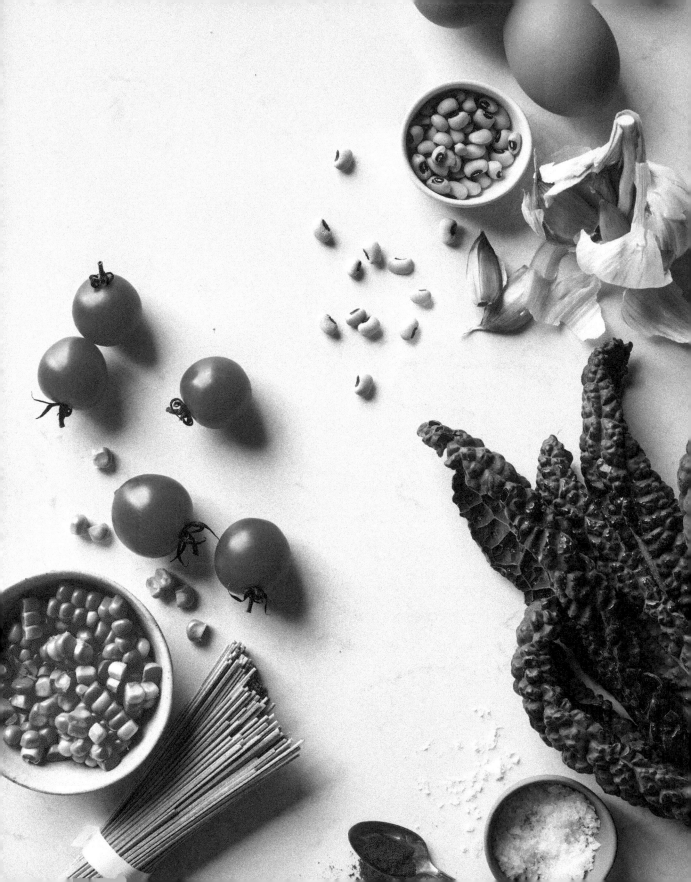

INTRODUCTION

If you picked up this book, there is a good chance you want to take control of your eating habits. Do you suspect that you eat too much sugar, but you don't know where to start to change that? Are you looking for better energy, a better mood, and to get control of cravings? If so, then you're in the right place.

Let me introduce myself. I'm a registered dietitian and food lover from Victoria, British Columbia, Canada. For 25 years, I've committed my life to helping people experience the good health that comes with eating healthy while still enjoying delicious food. I'm thrilled that you've picked up this cookbook, because now you too can experience the amazing benefits of eating real food without hidden sugar. As you will soon see, sugar is hiding everywhere, and it's having a big (negative) impact on your body. Kicking the sugar habit is one of the most significant actions that you can take to improve your health.

This cookbook is like an inside peek into how I teach my clients to eat without the travel expense of coming to my office in Victoria. Although, it is beautiful here, so you may still want to come for a visit! In case you're wondering, yes, this is how I eat, too. I didn't win the genetic lottery. Obesity, diabetes, heart conditions, high cholesterol, and early cancer all run in my family. I'm 40-something now and not only have I avoided all of these health concerns, I also have the energy to work 12-hour days in my own private practice, as well as surf, hike, trail run, and practice yoga. My intention is that, with this book, you too will find the health, happiness, and peace of mind that allows you to live your best life.

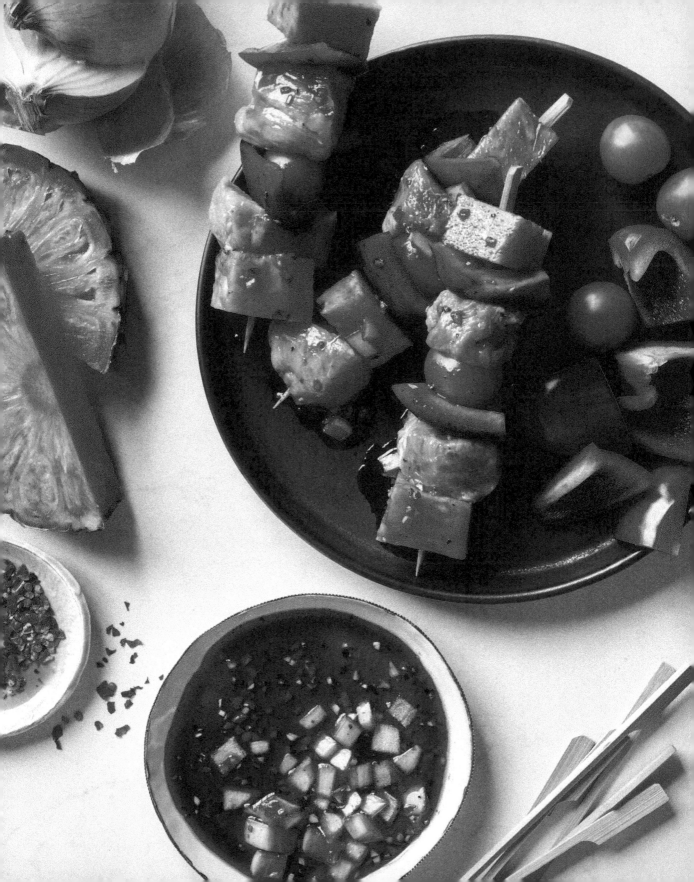

PART 1

Sugar Detox for Life

So, where is this book going? Chapter 1 breaks down what sugar is, chemically speaking, and what effect it has on our bodies. With your newfound understanding of the negative impact sugar is having on your body, you are empowered to do something about it. Chapter 2 has all the tools you need to kick the sugar habit for life—tools such as how to prevent cravings, how to spot the sugar hiding in foods, and how to plan meals now that you'll be cooking most of your food from scratch. In part 2, I share 125 recipes that are so delicious, they're sure to make you forget all about sugar. Let's get going.

1

THE NOT-SO-SWEET TRUTH ABOUT SUGAR

Sugar. Its sweet taste is undeniably delicious. But the unfortunate truth is that sugar's effect on our bodies isn't so sweet. In this chapter, we'll explore how our bodies process sugar, then uncover the tools needed to break the vicious cycle of sugar cravings, sugar highs, and sugar crashes.

Before we get into describing the effect that sugar has on your body, let's take a moment to define sugar. The word "sugar" can have a lot of different meanings, so this chapter establishes a clear definition.

What Is Sugar?

We all use the word "sugar," but what does it actually mean? Chemically speaking, a sugar is the simplest form of carbohydrate, only one or two units long. The single units are called monosaccharides, and the two-unit sugars are called disaccharides. In formal chemistry terms, the letters "-ose" are used to identify a sugar. You've likely heard of fructose, lactose, and glucose. You will often find these terms in the ingredient lists on food packages.

"Sugar" is the word used for the monosaccharides and disaccharides that occur naturally in foods and for the substance that is added to food. A number of foods naturally contain sugar, including milk, fruit, and some vegetables.

The food that we usually think of when we hear the word "sugar" is the white granular substance called "table sugar" or "white sugar." It is a disaccharide called sucrose made up of the monosaccharides glucose and fructose. Table sugar is made from either sugarcane or sugar beets. Note: Sugar beets are different than the beets we see in the supermarket. Sugar beets have specifically been bred to contain much, much more sugar than those beets. The following are all different forms of 100 percent sugar made from sugarcane (or sugar beets).

- Confectioners' sugar
- Brown sugar
- Demerara sugar
- Turbinado
- Muscovado sugar

- Raw sugar
- Molasses
- Liquid sugar
- Golden syrup
- Evaporated cane juice

These foods are also 100 percent sugar:

- Corn syrup
- Honey
- Maple syrup
- Agave

- Coconut sugar
- Date sugar
- Brown rice syrup

The term "free sugar" includes both the sugar that is added to foods, as well as the sugar naturally present in honey, syrups, and fruit juices. In this cookbook, we will be focusing on removing free sugars.

FRUCTOSE'S BAD RAP

From its presence in high-fructose corn syrup to the restriction of fruit in popular diets, fructose has had a lot of negative attention lately. But fructose doesn't fully deserve this bad reputation.

Fructose is found in a lot of foods. It is the monosaccharide that is naturally found in fruit, some vegetables, and honey. It is also found in the highly processed sugars refined from sugarcane and sugar beets (e.g., table sugar), as well as high-fructose corn syrup. Fructose is never found alone. It's always found in foods that also contain the sugars glucose and/or sucrose.

When research studies create very unnatural conditions, such as very high consumption levels of pure fructose, often in rats, they find significant negative health impacts, such as liver and kidney problems. However, when more realistic studies are done, with humans consuming real foods and drinks that have fructose, it's not possible to identify negative health effects that are unique to fructose. In the more realistic studies, the amount of fructose matters and the foods where you find the fructose matters. For example, eating fruits and vegetables is healthy, but drinking soda and other sugary drinks is unhealthy.

Bottom line: Blaming fructose is an oversimplification of the scientific research. What matters is how much sugar you consume and the foods that you eat. The healthy choice is to continue eating fruits and vegetables and to remove the free sugars from your diet.

What Happens When You Eat Sugar?

Now that we're on the same page about the meaning of the word sugar, let's discuss what happens in your body when you eat it. When eaten, sugar is absorbed into the blood and moved throughout our body to places like our liver, muscles, fat, and brain. In fact, all carbohydrates (carbs) are broken down in our intestines into individual sugars before they can start to be absorbed and circulated through our blood. The glycemic index (GI) is important when understanding the effect of sugar on our bodies. The GI ranks carbs on a scale from 0 to 100 based on how quickly they raise blood sugar after you eat. Foods with a high GI are digested quickly, causing a spike in blood sugar. Low GI carbs create more stable blood sugar.

After sugar has been absorbed into the blood, the hormone insulin is like a key opening the doors of the cells in our liver, our muscles, and our fat cells to let the sugar be transferred from the blood into these cells. Our brain uses sugar as its preferred fuel, and sugar is so important to the brain that it doesn't need insulin to unlock the door. Sugar crosses from our blood into our brain on its own.

Serotonin is nicknamed the "happy hormone" because it is related to mood. Most of our body's serotonin is found in our digestive tract and in our brain. Serotonin levels are low in people who have depression. It is known that low serotonin causes sugar cravings. Rat studies are being done to discover the exact relationship between sugar and serotonin. So far, it looks like a diet high in sugar may cause our bodies to be lazy about creating serotonin. Eating a lot of sugar makes you want to eat more sugar in order to maintain your serotonin levels and your mood.

The other happy chemical in our brain is dopamine. Dopamine is released when something good happens. It's also known as the reward chemical. Our brain likes dopamine to be released—it's part of the sensation of pleasure. When we eat sugar, dopamine is released, and we feel good. When the dopamine level comes back down, we crave more dopamine. In other words, we crave sugar. When we eat more sugar, the cycle starts all over again.

I call these effects of sugar on our bodies the blood sugar roller coaster. It's the cycle of spiking high and then crashing down. A key to having steady energy and a steady mood is to get off the blood sugar roller coaster.

IS IT POSSIBLE TO BE ADDICTED TO SUGAR?

This is such an important question, one that doesn't have a simple answer. Let me break it down for you. The first problem is that there are different definitions of addiction. The Canadian Mental Health Association identifies the four C's as a simple description of addiction:

1. Craving
2. Loss of Control of amount or frequency of use
3. Compulsion to use
4. Use despite Consequences

As you can see, if you use the four C's to define addiction, then yes, sugar addiction is very possible. However, the definitive guide to identifying mental health disorders, the *Diagnostic and Statistical Manual of Mental Disorders* (*DSM-V*), states that in addition to the four C's, addiction requires specific brain chemistry to be involved. Even though there is a lot of talk about sugar these days, there haven't been enough human studies done on the effects of sugar on our brain chemistry to determine the similarity or differences in the effects of sugar versus drugs or alcohol.

Bottom line: The current scientific evidence doesn't give a clear answer on the possibility of sugar being addictive.

Breaking the Cycle: Sugar Detox

As we covered in the last section, the key to feeling better is to break the blood sugar roller coaster, the cycle of blood sugar spikes and crashes. Breaking the cycle is the key to having steady energy and being free from cravings.

Congratulations! By picking up this cookbook, you've already taken the first step in kicking sugar to the curb.

The second step to breaking the cycle is very simple. You eliminate the free sugar from your diet: a sugar detox. When you eliminate free sugar, you won't have a sugar spike. Therefore, you won't have the sugar crash. The cycle comes to an end. Eliminating free sugar is like refusing to get on the roller coaster. Steady energy and control over cravings are the benefits you will experience.

In the next chapter, I give you the tools to get off (and stay off) the sugar cycle. Eating low sugar will be your new, sustainable lifestyle.

EIGHT WAYS TO FEEL FULL FAST

Feeling full is a complicated process. Our brain reads messages involving senses and signals within our stomach and intestine, communicated by nerves and hormones. It's like our brain is putting these pieces together to form a fullness puzzle. To make it even more complicated, our habits, emotions, and environment provide additional puzzle pieces.

Here are eight ways to feel full that target different puzzle pieces.

1. **Tune in. Multitasking while eating divides our attention. We don't register fullness as quickly when we're distracted by other actions, like driving or looking at screens (computer, TV, movies, phones, etc.).**
2. **Chew your food well. The act of chewing sends signals to your body to let it know that you've eaten, thus satisfying hunger.**
3. **Eat protein. Studies show that eating protein helps us feel full sooner.**
4. **Choose fiber. Fiber fills us up quickly and is found naturally in vegetables, fruit, nuts and seeds, beans and lentils, and real whole grains.**
5. **Include fat. Fat slows down our stomach emptying and sends fullness messages from our digestive tract to our brain.**
6. **Pick soup. Soup has a particular ability to make us feel full, as do other foods that naturally contain a lot of water, such as most fruits and vegetables.**
7. **Don't drink. Alcohol stimulates appetite.**
8. **Put less on your plate. The more food you put on your plate, the more you'll eat before you feel full.**

2

LIVING FREE OF FREE SUGAR

Are you tempted to jump right into the recipes? I'm excited for you to get to them, but do resist the temptation, at least for a moment. Recipes are important, but if you want to create your new, long-term lifestyle, this chapter is key. In this chapter, I share with you the essential tools you need for everyday sugar-free eating. I break down the lifestyle, step-by-step, so that you will be successful, even if you're not a great cook or have never prepped meals before. You'll also get all the names that free sugar hides under on food labels.

I know that you're going to love the freedom that these tools will give you. Welcome to your new lifestyle!

Good Riddance for Good Health

You're likely asking: "What foods are out, and what's in?" So, let's get into it.

Something that you'll notice about this cookbook is that I'm not removing whole foods that naturally contain sugar, such as fruit and dairy. A lot of other books make you remove these for a strict initial phase and then reintroduce them. However, I don't believe in restricting foods unnecessarily. Fruit and dairy foods aren't the problem. Free sugar is the real culprit, so we're focusing on removing it from your diet. As you're about to see, it's hiding in a lot more food than you realize.

Our taste buds are amazing. They adjust to the foods to which they're exposed. When we eat a lot of sugar, that level of sweetness becomes our "normal." I want to give your taste buds an opportunity to recalibrate. Once recalibrated, you will taste (and enjoy) the natural sweetness in whole foods, such as a red bell pepper. To allow your taste buds to adjust, I recommend avoiding artificial sweeteners or high-intensity sweeteners.

This list details which foods are in and which are out:

IN

- ✓ Vegetables (fresh, frozen, or canned)
- ✓ Fruit (fresh, frozen, or dried)
- ✓ Whole grain bread (bread made with whole wheat, whole grain rye, and rolled oats)
- ✓ Whole wheat pasta, brown rice pasta, and pasta made with beans (e.g., chickpea pasta)
- ✓ Grains (e.g., rice or quinoa)
- ✓ Cereal
- ✓ Nuts and seeds
- ✓ Beans and lentils
- ✓ Dairy (milk, cream, plain yogurt, cheese, or butter)
- ✓ Unsweetened plant-based dairy alternatives (e.g., almond milk)
- ✓ Meat
- ✓ Poultry
- ✓ Fish
- ✓ Soy foods (e.g., tofu or tempeh)
- ✓ Vegetable oils
- ✓ Vinegars
- ✓ Herbs and spices
- ✓ Tea, coffee (without free sugar or high-intensity sweeteners)
- ✓ Alcohol (without free sugar or high-intensity sweeteners)

OUT

- ✗ Sugar
- ✗ Honey
- ✗ Maple syrup
- ✗ Other sweeteners and syrups
- ✗ High-intensity sweeteners (artificial sweeteners)
- ✗ All foods that contain free sugar or high-intensity sweeteners, such as:
  - Breakfast cereal
  - Bread
  - Flavored yogurt
  - Canned soup
  - Prepackaged meals and side dishes
  - Frozen meals
  - Salad dressings, sauces, spreads, and condiments
  - Jam
  - Candy
  - Chocolate
  - Ice cream
  - Baking (e.g., cookies, cake, muffins, and pie)
  - Other confections
- ✗ Beverages that contain free sugar and high-intensity sweeteners:
  - Fruit juice
  - Soda
  - Diet soda
  - Fruit punch
  - Lemonade
  - Chocolate milk
  - Sweetened plant-based dairy alternatives (e.g., sweetened almond milk)
  - Sweetened hot or iced tea
  - Sweetened coffee
  - Alcohol containing free sugar

Keep It Complex to Curb the Cravings

As we discussed in What Happens When You Eat Sugar? (page 6), we feel better when we stay off the blood sugar roller coaster. Free sugar is the main culprit for these blood sugar spikes. However, refined carbohydrates can also cause quite a blood sugar spike. Other sugar detox books frequently remove all grains. However, whole grains don't cause the problematic blood sugar spike; in fact, they provide healthy fiber, vitamins, and minerals. Therefore, I recommend keeping them in your new lifestyle. While refined grains aren't officially "out," I recommend limiting them to an occasional meal. Perhaps you'll choose to go 100 percent whole grain. Perhaps you'll follow the 80/20 rule (80 percent whole grain to 20 percent refined grain). Choose the right balance for you.

This cookbook follows the 80/20 rule. There are lots of delicious whole grain recipes here. If brown rice just won't do and you have a hankering for white rice, give parboiled rice (also known as converted rice) a try. It's the lowest glycemic index of all the types of white rice. I've got delicious recipes for Peruvian Rice (page 180) and Spiced Rice and Peas (page 182).

Whole Grains

- Bread made with whole wheat, whole grain rye, and rolled oats
- Whole wheat and corn tortillas
- Whole wheat pasta, brown rice pasta, quinoa pasta, and chickpea pasta
- Brown rice
- Wild rice
- Quinoa
- Buckwheat (buckwheat groats)
- Barley
- Bulgur
- Steel cut and rolled oats
- Farro
- Amaranth

Learning to Shop Sugar Smart

Switching to a sugar-free lifestyle involves changing how you grocery shop. There are two key principles to shopping sugar smart:

1. Focus on food without labels: Many of the healthiest foods in the supermarket don't come with labels. I'm talking about foods like fresh fruit

and vegetables, meat, poultry, seafood, nuts, seeds, beans, and lentils. When foods are single ingredients like these, there is nowhere for free sugars or artificial sweeteners (high-intensity sweeteners) to hide.

2. **Read food labels:** Free sugar and high-intensity sweeteners are found in a lot of foods. Unfortunately, the "Sugars" listing in the nutrition facts panel doesn't differentiate between natural sugar (the good stuff) and free sugar (the bad stuff). For example, canned tomatoes will have 3 or 4 grams of sugar on the nutrition facts panel. That's the natural sugar within the tomatoes themselves. In this cookbook, we're focusing on removing only the unhealthy free sugars. Therefore, the nutrition facts panel doesn't give you the ability to differentiate between natural sugar and free sugar. For this reason, I don't recommend relying on it.

The ingredient list is where you'll find out whether a food contains free sugar or high-intensity sweeteners. The tricky thing is that many different words can be used to describe free sugar. Check out You Call It Maltitol, I Call It Sugar (page 16) for a list of words in ingredient lists that indicate free sugar and high-intensity sweeteners.

Start by reading the ingredient list of each packaged food that you are considering buying. While it will take some time in the beginning to read all of the food labels, soon you will find your go-to sugar-free foods, resulting in grocery shopping that's a breeze. In some cases, it is obvious that food contains free sugar or high-intensity sweeteners, such as with candy bars or ice cream. Some foods will be surprising, because they seem healthy. Be on the lookout for free sugars and high-intensity sweeteners in the following:

- Flavored yogurt
- Plant-based dairy alternatives (e.g., almond milk)
- "Healthy" breakfast cereals
- Bread
- Granola bars
- Canned fruit
- Peanut butter and other nut butters (e.g., almond butter)
- Condiments (e.g., ketchup)
- Salad dressing
- Pasta sauce
- Stir-fry sauce

YOU CALL IT MALTITOL, I CALL IT SUGAR

When reading the ingredient list on food labels, keep an eye out for these words, which all indicate free sugar or high-intensity sweeteners (also known as artificial sweeteners).

Free sugars
- "Sugar" with any descriptive word (e.g., confectioners' sugar, coconut sugar)
- Words ending in "-ose" (e.g., sucrose, glucose, glucose solids)
- "Syrup" with any descriptive word (e.g., brown rice syrup, corn syrup)
- Any phrase that contains the word "cane" (e.g., evaporated cane juice, cane juice crystals)
- Any phrase that contains the word "malt" (e.g., barley malt)
- Agave, agave nectar
- Caramel
- Corn sweetener
- Dextrin, maltodextrin
- Fruit juice
- Fruit juice concentrate

- HFCS (high-fructose corn syrup)
- Honey
- Maple syrup
- Molasses
- Muscovado
- Panocha
- Sweet sorghum
- Treacle

High-intensity sweeteners
- Words ending in "-ol" (e.g., xylitol, maltitol, sorbitol)
- Acesulfame potassium
- Advantame
- Aspartame
- Isomalt
- Neotame
- Saccharin
- Stevia
- Sucralose

Welcome to the Sugar Detox Kitchen!

As you can see, free sugar is hiding everywhere. The best way to avoid free sugar is to cook from scratch. New to cooking from scratch? You've got nothing to worry about. Everyone can cook. Yes, everyone. All it takes is a little planning and practice.

I've hand-selected the recipes in part 2 to be delicious (of course), but also to be simple for the beginner cook. They involve minimal prep, and they're made with easy-to-find ingredients. No long lists of rare ingredients; no recipes with 25 painstaking steps. First, I'll walk you step-by-step through the biggest secret to cooking from scratch. I'm talking about meal planning and meal prep. Welcome to the sugar detox kitchen—the home base of your new healthy lifestyle.

How to Plan a Week's Worth of Meals

There's nothing worse than arriving home hungry at the end of another long workday and staring blankly into the refrigerator, wondering what to make for dinner. The good news is that this daily stress can easily be prevented by doing a little planning.

Taking one hour to plan meals will save you time and stress all week long. Think of this time as an investment in your new lifestyle.

Here's a step-by-step guide to planning one week's worth of meals.

1. On a piece of paper/your computer/tablet/phone, create a table with space for every meal and snack listed by the day of the week. (See the Jump-Start Two-Week Sugar Detox Meal Plan on page 18 for inspiration.)

2. Open up your calendar. Identify what meals you plan to eat out (business lunches, dinner parties, etc). Identify what days you have more time to cook and what days will be a time crunch requiring quick, easy meals.

3. Check your refrigerator and pantry. What food do you already have that needs to be eaten before it goes bad? What meals do you have in the freezer that you can pull out on busy days, so you don't have to cook? What ingredients do you have in the cupboard that you can use for recipes?

4. Now it's time to write out your meal plan in this order:

- Refrigerated leftovers. Plan to eat these first so they don't go bad.
- Recipes involving refrigerated ingredients that won't keep for long, such as uncooked meat, poultry, or seafood. Also, vegetables, fruit, dairy, and deli meat.
- On days when you have more time to cook, choose dishes that take longer to prepare and cook.
- On time-crunch days, choose quick dishes.
- Fill in any remaining days. Look for opportunities for efficiency. For example, do you use only half a can of beans for a recipe on Monday? Choose a recipe for the second half of the can on Tuesday or Wednesday.

Jump-Start Two-Week Sugar Detox Meal Plan

Switching from eating a lot of free sugar to being sugar-free can feel intimidating—especially if you're used to eating out a lot and your version of eating in is ordering takeout or warming up a frozen dinner. But you've got nothing to fear. This cookbook has everything you need to jump-start your new sugar-free lifestyle.

The upcoming chapters have 125 delicious recipes that contain no free sugar. Here, I've created a two-week meal plan to show you how you can put them together to create your new lifestyle. This meal plan covers breakfast, lunch, and snacks for one person and dinners for two people. I've even provided grocery lists, so your trip to the supermarket is streamlined and you save money not buying things you don't need. Feel free to add desserts to this meal plan any day that you wish. Chapter 10 is full of recipes for delicious sweets that contain no free sugar. Just remember to add your dessert ingredients to your shopping list.

THE MAGIC OF MAKE AHEAD

There are days when you absolutely have no time to cook. And there are days when you arrive home completely exhausted and the last thing that you want to do is cook. These are the days when having prepared food waiting for you feels completely magical.

To tell you the truth, there isn't any magic to making that your reality. It's simply the result of planning. Here are some easy-to-implement make-ahead strategies:

- **Batch it.** On days when you have more time, make bigger batch meals. Refrigerate leftovers that you plan to use in the next two or three days. Freeze the rest in individual portions.

- **Use kitchen time efficiently.** Have 30 minutes to wait while dinner cooks in the oven? Use this time to cook up a batch of whole grain cereal for breakfasts for the next week or pre-portion snacks. You will see that we make strong use of the make ahead strategy in the **Jump-Start Two-Week Sugar Detox Meal Plan (page 18)**.

- **Make extra grains and beans.** Did you know that grains such as brown rice and quinoa freeze well? So do beans and lentils. When you cook these for one dish, make extra to freeze.

- **Chop extra.** Plan meals with similar ingredients several days in a row. If you're chopping up half a green pepper for dinner tonight, it only takes a moment longer to chop the other half for tomorrow's dinner. Or, if you need a carrot for dinner tonight, wash two carrots. Chop one carrot for tonight's dinner and cut the other one into carrot sticks for tomorrow's snack.

TWO-WEEK MEAL PLAN

	Breakfast	Lunch	Snack	Dinner	Make Ahead
MON	Pistachio-Mint Smoothie (page 30), served with 1 slice of whole grain toast	Toasted Mashed Bean and Avocado Sandwich (page 53), carrot sticks, and strawberries	Apple and a handful of almonds	Tomato-Ricotta Spaghetti (page 153)	Overnight Oats with Blueberries and Hemp Seeds (page 33)
TUE	Overnight Oats with Blueberries and Hemp Seeds (page 33)	Soba Noodle Salad (page 48)	Carrot sticks and a handful of pistachios	Fish Tacos	Hard-boil 6 eggs. Make Pink Pickled Eggs (page 34). Set aside some preshredded cabbage for Wednesday's snack.
WED	Pink Pickled Eggs (page 34), served with 1 slice of whole grain toast	Leftover Soba Noodle Salad	Slaw made from leftover preshredded cabbage, served with a handful of sunflower seeds	Sausage and Pepper Pasta (page 103)	Cook brown rice for Thursday dinner and Saturday lunch. Make White Bean Dip (page 71) using the remining white beans from the can you opened to make Monday's lunch.
THURS	Pink Pickled Eggs (page 34), served with 1 slice of whole grain toast	Leftover Sausage and Pepper Pasta	White Bean Dip (page 71), served with whole grain crackers and cherry tomatoes	Pork Lettuce Wraps (page 99), served with brown rice	Cut up an extra cucumber for Friday and Saturday snacks.
FRI	Pink Pickled Egg (page 34), served with 1 slice of whole grain toast	Leftover Sausage and Pepper Pasta	White Bean Dip (page 71), served with whole grain crackers and cucumber slices	Hamburgers with Hidden Veggies (page 111), served with a tossed salad	
SAT	Muffin Tin Mini Egg Frittatas (page 40), served with an orange	Leftover Pork Lettuce Wraps, served with brown rice	Apple-Cinnamon Muffin (page 79), served with a handful of almonds and cucumber slices	Seafood Cioppino (page 116), served with whole grain artisan bread and a tossed salad	
SUN	Buckwheat Pancakes with Almond Butter and Homemade Chunky Applesauce (page 42)	Leftover Hamburgers with Hidden Veggies, served with a tossed salad	Apple-Cinnamon Muffin (page 79), served with a handful of almonds and an apple	Lemon-Garlic Roast Chicken (page 91), served with Barley Tabouli (page 181) and half of the recipe for Swiss Chard with Capers and Raisins (page 173)	Fill the oven—roast a yam for Monday's lunch. Fill the oven—roast an eggplant and garlic for Monday's snack. Keep leftover chicken for Tuesday's dinner and Wednesday's lunch.

Shopping List Week 1

Fruits and Vegetables

- 7 apples
- 2 oranges
- 2 lemons
- 1 lime
- 2 avocados
- 1 head romaine lettuce
- 1 head Bibb lettuce
- 3 bunches spinach
- 1 bunch Swiss chard
- 1 bag preshredded cabbage (coleslaw mix)
- 10 carrots
- 2 green bell peppers
- 4 red bell peppers
- 2 yellow bell peppers
- 2 beets
- 4 English cucumbers
- 2 eggplants
- 6 tomatoes
- 5 cups grape or cherry tomatoes
- 1 yam
- 1 bunch fresh mint
- 1 bunch fresh dill
- 2 bunches fresh Italian flat-leaf parsley
- 1 bunch fresh cilantro
- 1 bunch fresh basil
- 1 bunch scallions
- 3 red onions
- 3 yellow onions
- 4 heads garlic
- 1 fresh ginger root
- 2 hot chile peppers (e.g., jalapeño)
- ½ cup unsweetened applesauce
- 1 (15-ounce) can whole baby beets
- 1 (28-ounce) can diced tomatoes
- 1 (15-ounce) can tomato sauce
- ½ cup frozen blueberries
- 1¼ cups raisins
- 3 dates

Starch Foods

- 12 ounces whole wheat spaghetti
- 12 ounces whole wheat rotini or penne
- 1 package soba noodles
- 1 loaf whole grain bread
- 1 loaf artisan whole grain bread
- 4 whole wheat hamburger buns
- Whole grain crackers
- 8 corn hard taco shells
- 2 cups brown rice
- ⅓ cup rolled oats
- 1 cup pearl barley
- 1 cup buckwheat flour
- 3½ cups whole wheat flour
- ½ cup all-purpose flour

Meat, Poultry, Seafood

- 1 pound ground pork
- 1 pound lean ground beef
- 4 Italian sausages
- 1 (3- to 4-pound) chicken, cut into 8 parts (2 breasts, 2 thighs, 2 legs, 2 wings)
- 2 pounds firm white fish (e.g., halibut, cod)
- 2 fillets tilapia
- 25 medium to large shrimp
- 25 mussels
- 1 (10-ounce) can clams

Dairy and Eggs

- 5 cups milk
- ⅓ cup plain yogurt
- 1½ cups cheddar cheese
- 2 cups ricotta cheese
- ¼ cup unsalted butter
- 1½ dozen large eggs

Vegetarian Proteins

- 1 cup sunflower seeds
- ¾ cup unsalted pistachios, shelled
- ½ cup walnuts
- ¼ cup hemp seeds
- ¼ cup sesame seeds
- ¼ cup salted peanuts
- 1 tablespoon ground flaxseed
- 1 jar unsweetened, natural almond butter
- 1 (15½-ounce) can white beans

Staples and Alcohol

- Cooking oil spray
- Extra-virgin olive oil
- Vegetable oil
- Sesame oil
- Balsamic vinegar
- Raw unfiltered apple cider vinegar
- White vinegar
- Rice vinegar
- Lemon juice
- Lime juice
- Soy sauce
- Mayonnaise
- Yellow mustard
- Hot sauce
- 1 small jar capers
- Ground black pepper
- Salt
- Coarse salt
- Pickling spice
- Dried oregano
- Dried basil
- Dried rosemary
- Paprika
- Cayenne
- Cinnamon
- Baking powder, baking soda
- 1 cup white wine

TWO-WEEK MEAL PLAN

	Breakfast	Lunch	Snack	Dinner	Make Ahead
MON	Muffin Tin Mini Egg Frittatas (page 40), served with strawberries	Smoked Tofu Wrap with Yams (page 54), served with an apple	Baba Ghanoush (page 66), served with whole grain crackers	Smokey Tempeh (page 147), served with Leftover Barley Tabouli and a tossed salad	
TUE	Buckwheat Pancakes with Almond Butter and Homemade Chunky Applesauce (page 42)	Leftover Seafood Cioppino, served with artisan whole grain bread and a tossed salad	Apple-Cinnamon Muffin (page 79), served with leftover Smokey Tempeh and an apple	Chicken Tacos (page 90)	Slice extra bell peppers for Wednesday's lunch, Overnight Oats with Blueberries and Hemp Seeds (page 33)
WED	Overnight Oats with Blueberries and Hemp Seeds (page 33)	Chicken Salad Sandwich with Apples, Grapes, and Walnuts (page 59), served with sliced bell peppers	Apple-Cinnamon Muffin (page 79), served with a handful of almonds and an apple	Caribbean Tofu (page 148), served with quinoa and Build Your Own Slaw (page 169)	Cook extra quinoa for Friday and Saturday lunches. While you're on a roll with quinoa, make Hot Quinoa Cereal with Dates and Coconut (page 36) for Thursday and Friday breakfasts.
THURS	Hot Quinoa Cereal with Dates and Coconut (page 36)	Smoked Tofu Wrap with Yams (page 54), served with an apple	Baba Ghanoush (page 66), served with whole grain crackers	Pan-Seared Steak with Carrot-Parsnip Mash (page 108)	
FRI	Hot Quinoa Cereal with Dates and Coconut (page 36)	Some Like It Hot Steak Salad (page 51)	Apple-Cinnamon Muffin (page 79), served with leftover Caribbean Tofu and an apple	Lemon-Garlic Shrimp Kebabs (page 118), served with Peruvian Rice (page 180) and Orange, Cucumber, and Jicama Salad (page 168)	Cook extra shrimp for Saturday snack and Sunday lunch.
SAT	Cinnamon-Raisin Whole Grain Cereal (page 37)	Leftover Some Like It Hot Steak Salad	Avocado Halves with Shrimp (page 82)	Chicken Cassoulet (page 93)	
SUN	Scrambled Tofu (page 39), served with whole grain toast and an orange	Shrimp Rice Paper Wraps (page 55)	Carrot Yogurt Dip (page 68), served with whole grain crackers	Jenefer's Chili Con Carne (page 104), served with brown rice	Make enough brown rice for leftovers next week.

Shopping List Week 2

Fruit and Vegetables

- 1 cup strawberries
- 6 apples
- 6 oranges
- 1 bunch red seedless grapes
- 3 lemon
- 2 limes
- 2 avocados
- 1 head romaine lettuce
- 1 head Bibb lettuce
- 1 bag preshredded cabbage (coleslaw mix)
- 4 English cucumbers
- 1 large jicama
- 12 carrots
- 4 parsnips
- 4 green bell peppers
- 3 red bell peppers
- 3 orange bell peppers
- 5 Roma tomatoes
- 1½ cups cherry or grape tomatoes
- 1 package pea shoots
- 1 celery stalk
- 1 bunch fresh parsley
- 1 bunch fresh cilantro
- 1 bunch scallions
- 2 red onions
- 2 yellow onions
- 3 heads garlic
- 4 hot chile peppers (e.g., jalapeño)
- 1 (28-ounce) can diced tomatoes
- 1 (6-ounce) can tomato paste
- ½ cup frozen blueberries
- ¼ cup raisins
- 3 dates

Starch Foods

- 3 cups quinoa
- 2 cups parboiled (converted) rice
- ½ cup buckwheat groats
- ½ cup bulgur
- ⅓ cup rolled oats
- 1 loaf whole grain bread
- 2 whole wheat tortilla wraps
- 8 corn hard taco shells
- Whole grain crackers
- 4½ ounces rice vermicelli or rice stick noodles
- 4 rice paper wraps

Meat, Poultry, Seafood

- 4 sirloin steaks, at least ¾-inch thick
- 1½ pounds lean ground beef
- ¾ pound kielbasa sausage
- 6 chicken drumsticks
- 52 medium or large shrimp

Dairy and Eggs

- 1¼ cups milk
- 1 cup plain, unsweetened Greek yogurt
- 1 small container sour cream or plain, unsweetened yogurt
- ¼ cup unsalted butter

Vegetarian Proteins

- 2 (14-ounce) packages extra-firm tofu
- 1 (14-ounce) package smoked tofu
- 1 (8-ounce) package tempeh
- ¼ cup hemp seeds
- ¼ cup sunflower seeds
- ¼ cup pistachios, unshelled
- 1 tablespoon walnut pieces
- 1 jar unsweetened, natural almond butter
- 1 jar smooth unsweetened, natural peanut butter
- 2 (15½-ounce) cans pinto beans
- 2 (15½-ounce) cans cannellini beans

Staples and Alcohol

- Extra-virgin olive oil
- Vegetable oil
- Balsamic vinegar
- Raw unfiltered apple cider vinegar
- Rice vinegar
- White wine vinegar
- Lemon juice
- Lime juice
- Soy sauce
- Mayonnaise
- Hot sauce
- 1 jar pickled hot banana pepper rings
- 1 jar salsa
- 1 can coconut milk
- Salt
- Ground black pepper
- Paprika
- Turmeric
- Thyme
- Bay leaves
- Cumin
- Chili powder
- Garlic powder
- Cayenne
- Cinnamon
- ⅓ cup unsweetened shredded coconut, medium-size
- 1 cup white wine

SOBA NOODLE SALAD, PAGE 48

PART 2

The Recipes

Here we go. It's finally the part that you've been waiting for: the recipes! As I mentioned previously, I've selected these recipes to be both delicious and simple for the beginner cook. You are covered all day long—from breakfast through dinner, and snacks, too. There are quick recipes for rushed weekdays. There are also recipes that take a bit longer, but they make a large amount of food. When you invest the hour or so to make these recipes, you will get not only dinner tonight but also meals for another day. Having guests over? There are simple, yet elegant, recipes that are perfect for entertaining.

3

BREAKFAST

WINTER VEGETABLE
SHAKSHUKA, PAGE 41

Pistachio-Mint Smoothie

VEGETARIAN, VEGAN (OPTION), GLUTEN-FREE

SERVES 1 / TOTAL TIME: 5 MINUTES

This light, refreshing smoothie is perfect on hot summer mornings. One sip will transport you back to that first time you tried pistachio ice cream or when that one friend ordered two scoops over a waffle cone and you thought, "Pistachio ice cream? Yuck!" But then you gave the green treat a lick and came to realize the deceptively sweet power of the little shelled nut. The mint in this recipe does a great job of bringing out pistachio's unique flavor.

1 cup fresh spinach

¾ cup milk or plant-based milk alternative (e.g., almond milk)

⅓ cup plain yogurt, coconut yogurt, or soy yogurt

3 tablespoons unsalted pistachios, shelled

3 dates, chopped

2 tablespoons (packed) fresh mint leaves

1 tablespoon ground flaxseed

Combine all the ingredients in a blender. Blend until smooth.

Time-saving tip: The night before, put all the ingredients in the blender and store in the refrigerator. In the morning, all you need to do is blend it up.

PER SERVING: Calories: 496; Total fat: 16g; Total carbohydrates: 78g; Fiber: 9g; Protein: 18g; Sodium: 172mg

HOW TO BUILD A BALANCED SMOOTHIE

Smoothies can be a handy breakfast choice on rushed mornings. But they can also be really high in sugar if you're not careful.

The formula for a balanced smoothie includes protein, up to 1 cup of fruit, a source of healthy fat, and a liquid that doesn't contain free sugars. The protein and fat will help you stay full until lunchtime. Limit fruit to 1 cup to make sure you don't spike your blood sugar. Two optional components are vegetables and whole grains. Veggies at breakfast is a great jump start on eating your daily target for vegetables. Whole grains will provide extra energy, and their fiber will help keep you full.

Here are examples of foods that provide each of the formula's components. You will notice that some foods play more than one role.

Protein
- Nuts and seeds (e.g., hemp seeds, pumpkin seeds)
- Natural, no-sugar added nut butters (e.g., peanut butter, almond butter)
- Protein powder, no-sugar added
- Plain yogurt
- Soft tofu
- Precooked lentils

Fruit
- Half a banana
- 1 cup fresh or frozen fruit (e.g., blueberries, diced mango)
- 3 dates

Healthy fat
- Nuts and seeds (e.g., ground flaxseed, chia seeds)
- ¼ avocado
- 1 teaspoon avocado oil
- 1 teaspoon flaxseed oil

Vegetables
- Fresh or frozen leafy greens (e.g., spinach, kale)
- Grated raw beet

Whole grains
- ¼ cup rolled oats
- ¼ cup precooked quinoa
- ¼ cup precooked amaranth

Liquid
- Milk
- Unsweetened, plant-based milk alternative (e.g., almond milk)
- Water

Chocolate-Apricot Not-Granola Parfait

VEGETARIAN, VEGAN (OPTION), GLUTEN-FREE, MAKES GREAT LEFTOVERS

SERVES 1 (MAKES 3 SERVINGS OF THE TOPPING) / TOTAL TIME: 5 MINUTES

While granola enjoys a reputation as a health food, it's loaded with free sugar. That's why I call this not-granola. It gives you the satisfying crunch of granola without all the free sugar. With the natural sweetness from the apricots and coconut and the intense chocolate flavor of the cacao nibs, you won't miss the free sugar.

FOR THE TOPPING

⅓ **cup slivered almonds**

⅓ **cup pumpkin seeds**

⅓ **cup hemp seeds**

5 dried apricots, diced

4 tablespoons cacao nibs

¼ **cup unsweetened coconut, medium shredded**

FOR THE PARFAIT

¾ **cup plain, unsweetened yogurt, coconut yogurt, or soy yogurt**

½ **banana, sliced**

TO MAKE THE TOPPING

In a mason jar or reusable plastic container, combine the almonds, seeds, apricots, cacao nibs, and coconut.

TO MAKE THE PARFAIT

In a serving bowl, mason jar, or plastic reusable container, put the yogurt. Top with banana and ½ cup of the topping mixture.

Ingredient tip: Tart cherries are a divine alternative to the dried apricots. They are more expensive and difficult to find, but cherries and chocolate are a match made in heaven. Another fun splurge is to use large flake coconut instead of the medium shredded coconut.

PER SERVING (INCLUDES ⅓ OF THE TOTAL TOPPINGS):
Calories: 335; Total fat: 15g; Total carbohydrates: 37g; Fiber: 7g; Protein: 12g; Sodium: 146mg

Overnight Oats with Blueberries and Hemp Seeds

VEGETARIAN, VEGAN (OPTION), GLUTEN-FREE (OPTION), MAKE AHEAD

SERVES 1 / PREP TIME: 3 MINUTES, PLUS SOAKING OVERNIGHT

Did you know that you don't have to cook oats before you eat them? You simply soak them overnight and, like magic, they're ready in the morning. Frozen fruit works well because it defrosts overnight and is ready to enjoy in the morning. This is a great recipe for rushed mornings. To take your oats on-the-go, prepare them the night before in a mason jar (with lid) or plastic storage container.

⅓ cup rolled oats (gluten-free, if desired)

¼ cup hemp seeds

½ cup blueberries (fresh or frozen)

¾ cup milk or plant-based milk alternative (e.g., almond milk)

1. In a serving bowl, combine the oats, hemp seeds, blueberries, and milk.
2. Stir to make sure the oats are saturated with the milk.
3. Put in the refrigerator.
4. Serve the next morning.

Ingredient tip: Mix it up. Swap out the blueberries for other fruits and swap out the hemp seeds for other seeds or nuts. Great combinations include raspberries with ground flaxseed, apples with walnuts, and mango with chia seeds.

PER SERVING: Calories: 441; Total fat: 21g; Total carbohydrates: 40g; Fiber: 9g; Protein: 23g; Sodium: 98mg

Pink Pickled Eggs

VEGETARIAN, GLUTEN-FREE, MAKE AHEAD, MAKES GREAT LEFTOVERS

SERVES 3 / ACTIVE TIME: 10 MINUTES / TOTAL TIME: 25 MINUTES (to account for cooling mixture before adding to jar), PLUS PICKLING OVERNIGHT

What do you imagine when you think about pickled eggs? A dusty jar filled with brine sitting behind a dim bar? Well, we're about to change that! These eggs are as pretty as they are delicious. They're a perfect grab-and-go breakfast when paired with some whole grain crackers and a piece of fruit. They also make a great snack or even part of a picnic lunch.

1 cup raw unfiltered apple cider vinegar

1 tablespoon coarse salt

1½ teaspoons pickling spice

3 garlic cloves, crushed with flat side of your knife

1 (15-ounce) can whole baby beets

1 red onion, quartered

4 sprigs fresh dill

6 hard-boiled eggs (see How to Make a Perfect Hard-Boiled Egg, page 35)

1. In a large saucepan, combine the vinegar, salt, pickling spice, and garlic. Bring to a simmer. Remove from the heat and let cool for 15 minutes.
2. Remove the beets from the can. Reserve the liquid.
3. In a 1-quart jar, layer the beets, red onion, dill, and eggs. Pour the cooled pickling liquid over the jar ingredients.
4. Measure the liquid from the can of beets. If needed, top with water to make 1 cup. Add to the pickled egg jar.
5. Cover the jar. Cool to room temperature, then transfer to the refrigerator. Refrigerate overnight.

Ingredient tip: You can use beets that you roast yourself instead of the canned ones here. Before putting them in the jar, remove the skins from your roasted beets and quarter them. Use 1 full cup of water to replace the canning liquid.

PER SERVING: Calories: 218; Total fat: 11g; Total carbohydrates: 13g; Fiber: 3g; Protein: 14g; Sodium: 2,346mg

HOW TO MAKE A PERFECT HARD-BOILED EGG

Green-gray yolks are a result of eggs cooking for too long. While there is nothing unhealthy about eating a hard-boiled egg with a green-gray yolk, it looks unappealing. Here's how to make a perfect hard-boiled egg:

1. Put eggs in a saucepan large enough that the eggs are in one layer and aren't touching each other. **You don't want to crowd the eggs.**

2. Add enough cold water so that the water is one inch above the eggs.

3. Over high heat, bring the water to a full rolling boil. **Immediately cover with a lid and remove from the heat. Set a timer and leave the eggs for 15 minutes.**

4. Place eggs in a colander and run under cold water.

5. Peel shells off eggs. **Gently roll the eggs back and forth on a countertop to fracture the shell before peeling.**

Hot Quinoa Cereal with Dates and Coconut

VEGETARIAN, VEGAN, GLUTEN-FREE, MAKES GREAT LEFTOVERS

SERVES 2 / PREP TIME: 5 MINUTES / COOK TIME: 20 MINUTES

Quinoa is unique in that it is a whole grain, but unlike most whole grains that take between 45 minutes to one hour to cook, it cooks in 20 minutes. I'll eat this dish hot on the first day that I make it, and then I like to eat it cold on subsequent mornings. To make a balanced meal, serve this cereal topped with your favorite nuts or seeds. I particularly like sunflower seeds.

½ cup quinoa

1½ cups water

3 dates, chopped

½ cup canned, full-fat coconut milk

½ teaspoon vanilla extract

⅓ cup unsweetened shredded coconut, medium size

1. In a small saucepan, combine the quinoa, water, and dates. Cover and bring to a boil over high heat. Reduce the heat to low and simmer for 20 minutes.

2. Add the coconut milk, vanilla, and shredded coconut. Stir to thoroughly combine. Heat for 1 minute, just until the coconut milk is warm.

Ingredient tip: Quinoa has a natural outer coating that tastes bitter. In the past, it was necessary to rinse quinoa before cooking it to remove this coating. The quinoa available in the supermarket now has been prerinsed so you don't need to do it.

PER SERVING: Calories: 454; Total fat: 22g; Total carbohydrates: 62g; Fiber: 7g; Protein: 8g; Sodium: 30mg

Cinnamon-Raisin Whole Grain Cereal

VEGETARIAN, VEGAN (OPTION), MAKES GREAT LEFTOVERS

SERVES 4 (LARGE SERVINGS) / COOK TIME: 25 MINUTES

This hearty cereal is made with two underappreciated whole grains. You can find buckwheat and bulgur (cracked wheat) in any supermarket with a good bulk food section. My Grannie would call this a stick-to-your-ribs breakfast—one that keeps you toasty and full on a dark, cold winter morning as you trudge through the snow (or icy rain) on your way to the next oasis of warmth.

4 cups water

½ cup buckwheat groats

½ cup bulgur

½ teaspoon cinnamon

½ cup milk or unsweetened plant-based milk alternative (e.g., almond milk)

¼ cup raisins

¼ cup sunflower seeds

1. In a large saucepan, combine the water with the buckwheat and bulgur. Cover and bring to a boil over high heat.
2. Reduce the heat to medium. Cook for 15 minutes, or until the water is absorbed and the grains are soft. Stir constantly, scraping the bottom to prevent sticking and burning.
3. Add the cinnamon and milk. Stir to combine. Heat for 3 to 5 minutes, until the milk is warmed.
4. Serve topped with raisins and sunflower seeds.
5. Refrigerate or freeze leftovers.

Ingredient tip: Mix and match your toppings. Instead of sunflower seeds and raisins, try fresh or frozen blueberries and slivered almonds or dried apricots and walnuts. If you like your cereal with more milk, add a splash of milk when serving.

PER SERVING: Calories: 231; Total fat: 5g; Total carbohydrates: 41g; Fiber: 5g; Protein: 8g; Sodium: 24mg

WAYS TO COMBAT CRAVINGS

Don't go too long without eating. It typically takes four hours to digest a balanced meal and start to become hungry again. When you go much longer than 4 hours, you start to get hungrier and hungrier. The hungrier you get, the more likely you'll choose highly processed foods containing lots of free sugar. So, the best way to combat cravings is to eat when you are just starting to get hungry, about every 4 hours.

Here's what to choose:

Eat fiber. Every time that you are hungry, you are opening yourself up to cravings. Fiber-rich foods keep you full. You'll find fiber in vegetables, fruit, whole grains, nuts and seeds, and beans and lentils.

Eat protein. Protein keeps us full for several hours. In addition, protein doesn't spike your blood sugar, so it helps to keep you off the blood sugar roller coaster. Include protein-rich foods at each meal and snacks, too. Foods high in protein include meat, poultry, seafood, beans and lentils, nuts and seeds, soy foods (e.g., tofu), yogurt, and cheese.

Eat fat. Fat is what keeps us full the longest and, like protein, it doesn't spike your blood sugar. Include fat at meals and snacks. Healthy fat sources include fish, nuts and seeds, avocados, olives, and olive oil.

Change your environment. Similar to that classic experiment by Pavlov in which the dogs became hungry when the bell rang, we get cravings in specific environments. For example, has your habit been to sit on the couch at the end of the day, watching TV and eating candy? To get rid of the craving, you need to change your environment. Instead of watching TV on the couch, sit in a different location and read a book. Go for a walk. Or go to bed early.

Scrambled Tofu

VEGETARIAN, VEGAN, GLUTEN-FREE

SERVES 1 / PREP TIME: 5 MINUTES / COOK TIME: 5 MINUTES

Tofu is not actually the mushy, white sponge that cartoons have long made it out to be. It's simply a blank canvas upon which you can create many a masterpiece. This is a delicious recipe that is reminiscent of savory scrambled eggs. To create a balanced meal, serve it with your favorite fruit and whole grain toast.

1 tablespoon vegetable oil

2 scallions, finely chopped

1 garlic clove, minced

⅓ (14-ounce) package extra-firm tofu

1 tablespoon water

¼ teaspoon paprika

¼ teaspoon turmeric

¼ teaspoon cumin

¼ teaspoon chili powder

¼ cup parsley, finely chopped

1. Heat the vegetable oil in a small sauté pan or skillet over medium heat. Add the scallions and garlic. Sauté for 2 minutes.
2. Using your fingers, crumble the tofu into the pan. Add the water, paprika, turmeric, cumin, and chili powder, stirring to mix. Sauté for 2 minutes.
3. Add the parsley, stirring to mix. Sauté for 30 seconds more.
4. Serve immediately.

Ingredient tip: Medium-firm tofu and firm tofu also work well in this recipe. They will result in a softer-textured dish. Medium-firm tofu has a texture similar to soft scrambled eggs, while the extra-firm tofu called for here has a texture similar to eggs scrambled hard or well-done.

PER SERVING: Calories: 274; Total fat: 21g; Total carbohydrates: 11g; Fiber: 4g; Protein: 15g; Sodium: 38mg

Muffin Tin Mini Egg Frittatas

VEGETARIAN, GLUTEN-FREE, MAKES GREAT LEFTOVERS

MAKES 12 FRITTATAS / PREP TIME: 10 MINUTES / COOK TIME: 15 MINUTES, PLUS 5 MINUTES TO REST

Any recipe that involves veggies at breakfast makes this dietitian happy. These are an irresistible, hot make-ahead breakfast. Simply freeze in individual portions, defrost in the refrigerator the night before, then reheat in the microwave in the morning. Having a breakfast like this ready for you on rushed mornings will fill you up, thus saving you from the temptation of stopping at the coffee shop for a sugar-filled pastry.

Cooking oil spray

6 large eggs

½ cup milk

¼ teaspoon salt

¼ teaspoon black pepper

1 teaspoon dried oregano

¼ cup fresh parsley, chopped

2 scallions, finely chopped

1 red bell pepper, diced

2 cups spinach, coarsely chopped

1 cup cheddar, shredded

1. Preheat the oven to 375°F.
2. Spray a muffin tin with a generous amount of cooking oil spray, being sure to coat both the bottom and sides of each muffin cup.
3. Whisk together the eggs, milk, salt, pepper, and oregano. Add in the parsley, scallions, and red bell pepper.
4. Divide the spinach evenly and add to the bottom of each muffin cup. Pour in the egg mix, dividing it evenly among the cups. Top with the shredded cheese.
5. Bake 12 minutes, or until the egg is cooked through.
6. Allow to rest 5 minutes. Run a knife around the edge of each cup to loosen the egg, then pop it out.

Ingredient tip: Mix and match your veggies in this recipe. Mushrooms, baby kale, and Spanish (red) onion are just a few other vegetables that pair well with eggs.

PER SERVING (1 FRITTATA): Calories: 85; Total fat: 6g; Total carbohydrates: 2g; Fiber: 0g; Protein: 6g; Sodium: 153mg

Winter Vegetable Shakshuka

VEGETARIAN, GLUTEN-FREE

SERVES 1 / PREP TIME: 25 MINUTES / COOK TIME: 10 MINUTES

I was first introduced to shakshuka while travelling to a small village on an island that is a part of India and is popular among young Israeli travelers. While I'm sure that the version that I ate on that remote island was far from traditional, it was delicious. Since then, I've continued to make my spin on this dish using different local vegetables. Having a friend over for brunch? You can easily double the recipe and impress them with this unique meal. You can even quadruple the eggs (i.e., serving 4 people) but you likely won't need four times the veggies.

1 tablespoon extra-virgin olive oil

1 cup sliced leek, whites only (1 leek)

1 garlic clove, minced

1 cup mushrooms, sliced

1 cup rutabaga, shredded

⅛ teaspoon salt

⅛ teaspoon ground black pepper

2 cups spinach, roughly chopped and packed

2 large eggs

Hot sauce (optional)

1. In a small saucepan with a lid, heat the oil over medium heat. Add the leek, garlic, mushrooms, rutabaga, salt, and pepper. Cook for 5 minutes, stirring.
2. Add the spinach, in batches if needed. Cook until just wilted.
3. Make two small nests in the vegetables. Crack an egg into each nest. Reduce the heat to low-medium. Cover and cook until the whites are set and yolks runny, about 3 minutes.
4. Top with hot sauce (if using), and serve immediately.

Time-saving tip: A food processor fitted with a shredding blade makes quick work of the rutabaga.

PER SERVING: Calories: 428; Total fat: 24g; Total carbohydrates: 32g; Fiber: 8g; Protein: 20g; Sodium: 702mg

Buckwheat Pancakes with Almond Butter and Homemade Chunky Applesauce

VEGETARIAN, GLUTEN-FREE (OPTION), MAKES GREAT LEFTOVERS

SERVES 4 / PREP TIME: 10 MINUTES / COOK TIME: 20 MINUTES

This weekend morning recipe encompasses all the earthy flavors of fall. Throw on your flannel, pop a pumpkin on your porch, break out your favorite spooky movies, and get ready to experience autumn on your taste buds. This is a great recipe to turn to when those November apple pie cravings kick in. It's also a great recipe when you're craving breakfast-for-dinner. For the applesauce, I like to leave the skin on for extra fiber and texture, but you can peel the apples, if you prefer.

FOR THE APPLESAUCE

2 apples, cored and diced

1 cup water

FOR THE PANCAKES

1 cup buckwheat flour

1 cup whole wheat flour (gluten-free flour, if desired)

2 teaspoons baking powder

½ teaspoon salt

2 eggs, beaten

2 cups milk

3 tablespoons vegetable oil, divided

Natural almond butter (unsweetened)

TO MAKE THE APPLESAUCE

1. In a large saucepan, combine the diced apple with the water. Bring to a boil over high heat.
2. Lower the heat to medium and cook, stirring frequently, until the apples are soft and the water has evaporated, with some apple chunks remaining. Add extra water if it evaporates before the apples are soft.
3. Remove from the heat and allow to cool.

TO MAKE THE PANCAKES

1. In a large bowl, combine the flours, baking powder, and salt. Stir to mix thoroughly.
2. In a medium bowl, combine the eggs, milk, and 1 tablespoon of the oil.
3. Add the wet mixture to the dry ingredients. Stir to combine, making sure there are no lumps.

4. Heat a skillet over medium to medium-high heat. Add the remaining vegetable oil. When the oil is hot, spoon the batter into the pan, forming pancakes the size you desire. Flip the pancakes when bubbles rise up through the batter. Cook until the second side has browned.
5. Place the pancakes on a plate lined with a paper towel to absorb any excess oil.
6. Cook the remaining batter in batches. Refresh the vegetable oil in the skillet as needed.
7. Serve topped with almond butter and applesauce.
8. Refrigerate or freeze leftovers.

Equipment tip: An electric griddle also works well for cooking these pancakes.

PER SERVING: Calories: 435; Total fat: 16g; Total carbohydrates: 64g; Fiber: 10g; Protein: 15g; Sodium: 388mg

4

LUNCH

TOMATO, BLACK BEAN,
AND CORN SALAD, PAGE 46

Tomato, Black Bean, and Corn Salad

VEGETARIAN, VEGAN, MAKE AHEAD, MAKES GREAT LEFTOVERS

SERVES 2 / TOTAL TIME: 15 MINUTES

This refreshing salad bowl is light enough to enjoy on a summer day, but with black beans and brown rice, it satisfies as a full meal. The classic Mexican-inspired combination of rice and beans with bell peppers, tomatoes, avocado, and cilantro are paired with a dressing tasting of citrus, cumin, and coriander. You'll recognize these familiar flavors, and you'll enjoy them in this refreshing twist as a vegan salad.

FOR THE SALAD

1 (15½-ounce) can black beans, drained and rinsed

1 cup kernel corn, fresh, frozen, or canned

1 cup cooked brown rice

2 tomatoes, diced

1 avocado, diced

1 orange bell pepper, diced

1 yellow bell pepper, diced

1 bunch fresh cilantro

1 bunch fresh flat-leaf parsley

FOR THE DRESSING

3 tablespoons lime juice

2 tablespoons avocado oil

1 tablespoon white wine vinegar

1 tablespoon lemon juice

½ teaspoon cumin

¼ teaspoon coriander

¼ teaspoon ground black pepper

⅛ teaspoon salt

1. In a large bowl, combine all the salad ingredients.
2. In a jar with a tight-fitting lid, combine all the dressing ingredients. Cover and shake.
3. Drizzle the dressing on the salad and toss to evenly distribute.

Storage tip: If you are planning to eat half the recipe today and save the second half for later, portion out today's salad before adding the avocado, cilantro, parsley, and the dressing. Add these ingredients fresh to the salad the day you intend to eat it.

PER SERVING: Calories: 708; Total fat: 30g; Total carbohydrates: 95g; Fiber: 24g; Protein: 21g; Sodium: 196mg

Lentil and Brown Rice Salad

VEGETARIAN, VEGAN, GLUTEN-FREE, MAKE AHEAD, MAKES GREAT LEFTOVERS

SERVES 2 / TOTAL TIME: 15 MINUTES

Lentils are often overlooked. Many people who find beans gassy can digest lentils with no problems. Here, lentils combine with brown rice and other veggies to make an earthy, filling salad bowl. The raisins and almonds provide the sweetness and crunch necessary for any great salad. I enjoy this salad year-round. I know that you will, too.

FOR THE SALAD

4 cups water

10 asparagus spears

1 (15½-ounce) can lentils, drained and rinsed

1 cup cooked brown rice

2 cups grated carrot

1 cup grated beet

¼ cup slivered almonds

¼ cup raisins

FOR THE DRESSING

¼ cup extra-virgin olive oil

2 tablespoons Dijon mustard

2 tablespoons balsamic vinegar

1. In a medium saucepan, bring the water to a boil.
2. Snap the tough ends off the asparagus. Add the asparagus to the boiling water. Cook until just tender, 3 minutes for thin asparagus, 5 minutes for thick asparagus. Immediately put the asparagus in a medium bowl filled with ice water.
3. In a second medium bowl, combine the lentils, brown rice, grated carrot, grated beet, asparagus, almonds, and raisins.
4. In a jar with a tight-fitting lid, combine the dressing ingredients. Shake to mix. Pour over the salad, tossing to coat the salad evenly.

Ingredient tip: Rinsing canned beans and lentils removes some of the molecules that make them gassy. Always take the time to thoroughly rinse canned beans and lentils for any recipe.

PER SERVING: Calories: 769; Total fat: 37g; Total carbohydrates: 92g; Fiber: 22g; Protein: 23g; Sodium: 501mg

Soba Noodle Salad

VEGETARIAN, VEGAN, MAKES GREAT LEFTOVERS

SERVES 2 / TOTAL TIME: 20 MINUTES

This full-meal salad bowl is the perfect balance of textures and tastes, with crunchy sunflower seeds, toothsome shredded carrot and beets, silky noodles, creamy avocado, and chewy raisins. It's a salad that even non-salad eaters enjoy—including kids. I've turned many a picky kid into a salad eater with this recipe. If you can't find soba noodles, use whole wheat spaghetti noodles, cut in half.

FOR THE SALAD

1 bundle soba noodles

2 cups shredded carrots

2 cups shredded beets

1 avocado, diced

½ cup sunflower seeds

½ cup raisins

FOR THE DRESSING

3 tablespoons balsamic vinegar

1 tablespoon extra-virgin olive oil

¼ teaspoon ground black pepper

⅛ teaspoon salt

1. In a medium saucepan, bring water to a boil. Add the noodles. You may need to lower the heat to prevent boiling over. Boil for 5 minutes, until the noodles are al dente.

2. Strain the noodles into a colander and rinse under cold water until the noodles are cool to the touch.

3. In a medium bowl, combine the noodles, carrots, beets, avocado, seeds, and raisins.

4. In a jar with a lid, combine the dressing ingredients. Shake well to combine.

5. Pour the dressing over the salad, tossing to evenly coat the salad.

Ingredient tip: Soba noodles are a staple ingredient in Japanese cuisine. You can find them in any supermarket with a good Asian food section. Inside the package, the noodles come in neat bundles tied with little strips of paper.

PER SERVING: Calories: 760; Total fat: 37g; Total carbohydrates: 103g; Fiber: 17g; Protein: 18g; Sodium: 957mg

Classic Cobb Salad

GLUTEN-FREE, MAKE AHEAD

SERVES 1 / TOTAL TIME: 10 MINUTES

The secret to this salad is the planning. It's a decadent and quick lunch when you have your bacon, hard-boiled egg, and chicken all precooked. Serving guests? Simply double or quadruple the recipe—just make sure you check out How to Make a Perfect Hard-Boiled Egg (page 35).

FOR THE SALAD

3 romaine leaves, torn into bite-size pieces

¾ cup cherry or grape tomatoes, halved

1 hard-boiled egg, peeled and roughly chopped

¼ avocado, diced

2 pieces bacon, cooked and cut into bite-size pieces

1 cooked chicken breast, diced

2 tablespoons blue cheese, crumbled (optional)

FOR THE DRESSING

1 tablespoon shallot, finely diced

2 tablespoons apple cider vinegar

2 tablespoons extra-virgin olive oil

1 teaspoon Dijon mustard

1 pinch salt

1. Put the romaine lettuce in a large bowl and top with the remaining salad ingredients.
2. In a jar with a tight-fitting lid, combine all of the dressing ingredients. Cover and shake.
3. Drizzle the dressing on the salad and toss to evenly distribute.

Storage tip: If doubling this recipe to make leftovers, divide the portions before you add the avocado and dress the salad. Add diced avocado and dress the salad the day you plan to eat it.

PER SERVING: Calories: 627; Total fat: 49g; Total carbohydrates: 12g; Fiber: 5g; Protein: 39g; Sodium: 856mg

Chicken and Barley Greek Salad

MAKE AHEAD, MAKES GREAT LEFTOVERS

SERVES 2 / TOTAL TIME: 10 MINUTES

This salad combines the classic ingredients of a Greek salad with chicken breast and barley to make it a complete meal. It's a hearty enough salad to enjoy all year round. The next time that you're cooking chicken breast for dinner, make two extra breasts to enjoy for this salad. Or, use leftovers from Lemon-Garlic Roast Chicken (page 91). Barley takes time to cook, so when you make some, cook extra and freeze it. You can store barley in the freezer for 2 or 3 months.

FOR THE SALAD

2 cups cooked barley

1½ cups cherry or grape tomatoes, halved

1½ cups cucumber, diced

1 cup red onion, diced

2 cooked chicken breasts, diced

1 cup feta cheese, crumbled

12 kalamata olives

FOR THE DRESSING

2 tablespoons white wine vinegar

2 tablespoons lemon juice

1 tablespoon extra-virgin olive oil

1 teaspoon dried oregano

¼ teaspoon ground black pepper

1. In a large bowl, combine all the salad ingredients.
2. In a jar with a tight-fitting lid, combine all the dressing ingredients. Cover and shake.
3. Drizzle the dressing on the salad and toss to evenly distribute.

Prep tip: To cook the barley, combine 1 cup barley and 2 cups water in a small saucepan. Over high heat, cover and bring to a boil. When it comes to a boil, reduce the heat to low. Cook for 45 minutes, or until the water is absorbed and the barley is cooked.

PER SERVING: Calories: 690; Total fat: 33g; Total carbohydrates: 64g; Fiber: 10g; Protein: 40g; Sodium: 1,396mg

Some Like It Hot Steak Salad

GLUTEN-FREE, MAKE AHEAD, MAKES GREAT LEFTOVERS

SERVES 2 / TOTAL TIME: 10 MINUTES

It's worth cooking an extra steak for dinner in order to make this unique salad the next day. If you don't like spicy food, this salad also works without the pickled hot banana pepper rings (and the liquid from the jar). Really like to feel the burn? Toss more banana pepper rings into your salad and add more jar liquid to the dressing.

FOR THE SALAD

4 romaine lettuce leaves

1 cup cooked quinoa

1 (6-ounce) cooked steak, sliced,
(see Pan Seared Steak, page 108)

½ red onion, thinly sliced

1 cup cherry or grape
tomatoes, halved

1 cup diced cucumber

4 tablespoons pickled hot
banana pepper rings

FOR THE DRESSING

2 tablespoons
extra-virgin olive oil

½ cup cherry tomatoes, halved

3 tablespoons lime juice

1 teaspoon liquid from the jar of
pickled hot banana pepper rings

4 hot banana pepper rings

Pinch salt

1. Put the romaine lettuce in a large bowl and top with the remaining salad ingredients.
2. Combine all the dressing ingredients in a blender and purée.
3. Drizzle the dressing on the salad and toss to evenly distribute.

Prep tip: Here's a tip to release more juice from a lime. Before you cut them open, roll the limes on the kitchen counter, giving considerable pressure under the heel of your hand. Then, cut the limes in half and juice.

PER SERVING: Calories: 542; Total fat: 30g; Total carbohydrates: 43g; Fiber: 5g; Protein: 26g; Sodium: 909mg

Toasted Hummus Garden Sandwich

VEGETARIAN, VEGAN, GLUTEN-FREE (OPTION), MAKES GREAT LEFTOVERS

MAKES 1 SANDWICH / TOTAL TIME: 20 MINUTES

Hummus is a fantastic base for a sandwich piled high with veggies. You can mix and match the veggies in this sandwich—the list of veggies that will work well in it is almost endless. Examples include cucumber ribbons, roasted red pepper, and lettuce. Hummus is a very personal dish—everyone likes theirs with a little different balance of flavors. Enjoy strong garlic? Add a second clove. Enjoy lemony foods? Add more lemon juice. All the ingredients can be adjusted. This recipe makes enough hummus for snacks or a second set of sandwiches.

FOR THE HUMMUS

1 (15½-ounce) can chickpeas

¼ cup extra-virgin olive oil

¼ cup lemon juice
(fresh or bottled)

¼ cup tahini (sesame
seed butter)

1 garlic clove, minced

¼ teaspoon salt

FOR THE SANDWICH

2 pieces whole grain bread
(gluten-free, if desired)

¼ cup pea shoots

¼ cup grated carrot

¼ cup grated beet

1 tomato, sliced

1. Drain the chickpeas and rinse well.
2. In a blender, combine the chickpeas, olive oil, lemon juice, tahini, garlic, and salt. Blend until smooth.
3. Toast the bread. Assemble the sandwich.

Ingredient tip: Store-bought hummus also works well in this sandwich. Check the ingredient list to make sure it doesn't contain any free sugar.

PER SERVING (1 SANDWICH; 1 SERVING HUMMUS): Calories: 608; Total fat: 27g; Total carbohydrates: 80g; Fiber: 20g; Protein: 24g; Sodium: 632mg

PER SERVING (1 SERVING HUMMUS ONLY; 4 SERVINGS PER RECIPE): Calories: 331; Total fat: 23g; Total carbohydrates: 24g; Fiber: 7g; Protein: 9g; Sodium: 168mg

Toasted Mashed Bean and Avocado Sandwich

VEGETARIAN, VEGAN (OPTION), GLUTEN-FREE (OPTION)

MAKES 1 SANDWICH / TOTAL TIME: 5 MINUTES

This super-speedy sandwich is my go-to lunch on a busy day. It works best toasted, because the toast's texture is a good contrast with the avocado and mashed beans. Don't have access to a toaster at lunchtime? This sandwich works well as a wrap, too. Choose corn or whole wheat tortillas without added free sugar. Feel free to add your own toppings—lettuce, grated beet, carrot, and sprouts all work well here.

**2 pieces whole grain bread
(gluten-free, if desired)**

**½ cup white beans (e.g.,
cannellini beans)**

**1 tablespoon mayonnaise
(or vegan mayonnaise)**

**3 dashes hot sauce,
such as Tabasco**

Pinch salt

¼ avocado, sliced

1. Toast the bread.
2. In a small bowl, combine the beans, mayonnaise, hot sauce, and salt. Mash with a fork.
3. Assemble the sandwich by layering the bean mix on the toast and topping with the sliced avocado.

Ingredient tip: Any kind of bean works well in this sandwich. It's a fantastic way to use up any leftover beans (or lentils) from other recipes.

PER SERVING: Calories: 492; Total fat: 20g; Total carbohydrates: 69g; Fiber: 20g; Protein: 20g; Sodium: 568mg

Smoked Tofu Wrap with Yams

VEGETARIAN, VEGAN, GLUTEN-FREE (OPTION), MAKE AHEAD

MAKES 2 WRAPS / TOTAL TIME: 10 MINUTES, PLUS ABOUT 1 HOUR TO COOK THE YAM

Are you bored with your usual sandwiches? Change up your packed lunch with this totally different wrap. The natural sweetness from the yams and smoky tofu are a match made in heaven. Don't be turned off by the long cooking time. For packed lunches on busy weekday mornings, cook the yam the night before.

FOR THE YAM

1 yam

1 teaspoon extra-virgin olive oil

FOR THE WRAP

2 whole wheat wraps (gluten-free, if desired)

2 leaves romaine lettuce

½ (14-ounce) package smoked tofu

Dash cayenne

½ teaspoon cumin

½ cup pea shoots

4 inches from an English cucumber, cut into matchsticks

TO COOK THE YAM

1. Preheat the oven to 375°F.
2. Pierce the yam all over with a fork. Pour the oil in the center of a piece of aluminum foil large enough to wrap the yam. Roll yam in the oil to fully coat. Wrap the foil around the yam. Put in a metal or ceramic baking dish, fold-side up. Bake until soft, about 45 minutes. The baking time will depend on the size of your yam.
3. Allow to cool.

TO MAKE THE WRAP

1. Lay the two wraps on a flat surface. Place romaine lettuce on each wrap.
2. Divide the tofu into 6 slices. Place 3 pieces in the center of each wrap.
3. Remove the cooked yam from its skin and put in a small bowl. Mash. Add the cayenne and cumin and mix together. Spoon the yam over the tofu.
4. Add the pea shoots and cucumber and roll up the wrap.

Ingredient tip: You can find smoked tofu in the same section as the other tofu in your supermarket.

PER SERVING (1 WRAP): Calories: 461; Total fat: 14g; Total carbohydrates: 64g; Fiber: 11g; Protein: 32g; Sodium: 869mg

Shrimp Rice Paper Wraps

VEGAN (OPTION), GLUTEN-FREE

MAKES 4 WRAPS / TOTAL TIME: 30 MINUTES

It takes a few attempts to perfect the rolling technique for these wraps, but their bright flavor is worth the effort. Don't be tempted to put more than one rice paper wrap at a time in the water. They'll only stick together—I learned this one the hard way. You can find rice paper wraps in any supermarket with a good Asian food section. For a delicious vegan option, substitute roasted peanuts for the shrimp.

4½ ounces rice vermicelli or rice stick noodles

1 teaspoon salt

16 medium or large shrimp, deveined

4 scallions

1 carrot

1 English cucumber

¼ cup smooth natural peanut butter (unsweetened)

3 tablespoons rice vinegar (unseasoned)

2 teaspoons lime juice

3 teaspoons water

4 rice paper wraps

8 sprigs fresh cilantro

1 lime, quartered

1. Bring a large pot, preferably a double boiler, of water to a boil. Add the noodles. Cook for 3 or 4 minutes, until soft (rice stick noodles will take 1 or 2 minutes longer). Drain and rinse with cold water.

2. If you used a double boiler for the noodles, return the same pot of water to a boil. If you don't have a double boiler, bring a pot of fresh water to a boil.

3. While waiting for the water to boil, cut the green tops from the white bottoms of the scallions.

4. When the water boils, add the salt and shrimp and lower the heat to medium-high to prevent boiling over. Cook about 3 to 5 minutes, until the shrimp are cooked. Drain the shrimp and put them in a bowl of very cold water. When cool, remove the shells and tails from the shrimp.

5. Using a sharp vegetable peeler, peel the carrot and cucumber, then cut them into long ribbons. If you have a particularly juicy cucumber, put the ribbons in a bowl lined with a paper towel.

6. To make the sauce, in a small bowl, combine the peanut butter, vinegar, and lime juice. Stir well to combine. Add the water, ½ tablespoon at a time, until a sauce consistency is reached.

Continued

7. Create an assembly line of all the ingredients.
8. Half-fill a large, wide bowl with very hot (not boiling) water. Place one rice paper wrap in the bowl for a few seconds until pliable.
9. Working quickly, place the wrap on a flat work surface. In the center of the wrap, place the noodles, cucumber, carrot, scallion, and cilantro, making a bed for the shrimp. Place 4 shrimp per wrap on top of the veggies. Top with peanut sauce and a squeeze of fresh lime juice. Tuck up the bottom of the wrap, then roll.
10. Repeat for the 3 remaining wraps.

Ingredient tip: Reserve the white part of the scallions for another recipe. For example, they're great in a stir-fry or Muffin Tin Mini Egg Frittatas (page 40).

PER SERVING (1 WRAP): Calories: 307; Total fat: 9g; Total carbohydrates: 41g; Fiber: 4g; Protein: 16g; Sodium: 1,054mg

Homemade California Roll with Brown Rice

GLUTEN-FREE (OPTION), MAKE AHEAD

MAKES 4 SUSHI ROLLS / TOTAL TIME: 90 MINUTES

Don't be intimidated by sushi. California rolls are the perfect choice for the beginner to make at home because they don't contain any raw fish. This is a fun recipe to make for a cooking date or as an activity with a group of friends. You can find nori (the sheets of roasted seaweed), rice vinegar, pickled ginger, and wasabi in any supermarket with a good Asian food section. To make this recipe faster, prepare the brown rice ahead of time.

1 cup brown rice

2 cups water

4 teaspoons rice vinegar (unseasoned)

⅛ teaspoon salt

1 avocado

1 cucumber, English variety preferred

4 sheets nori (roasted seaweed)

1 can crabmeat

Mayonnaise

Pickled ginger (optional)

Reduced-sodium soy sauce (or gluten-free tamari, if desired, optional)

Wasabi (optional)

1. In a large saucepan, combine the rice and water. Cover and bring to a boil over high heat. When it boils, reduce the heat to low and cook until the water is evaporated, about 45 minutes.

2. When the rice is cooked, spread it out in a shallow dish. Add the rice vinegar and salt. Mix thoroughly. Allow to cool completely.

3. Cut the avocado into long strips. Peel the cucumber. If you are using a field cucumber, remove the seeds. Measure the cucumber beside a sheet of nori and cut it to the length of the nori. Then, cut the cucumber lengthwise into long, half-inch-wide rectangular strips.

4. On a flat surface, put 1 piece of nori.

5. Using wet hands, press an even layer of rice over the nori, leaving a ½ inch of bare nori along one edge.

6. Place one cucumber strip in the middle of the nori, in the same direction as your bare edge. Place a line of avocado alongside the cucumber. Place a line of crabmeat alongside the cucumber and avocado.

7. Top the crabmeat with a line of mayonnaise.

Continued

8. Run a wet finger along the edge of the nori to dampen it. Quickly (before the damp edge dries), roll up the nori, tightly, from the full edge toward the wet edge. Using the wet edge like glue to seal the sushi roll.
9. Cut into round pieces.
10. Repeat with the remaining 3 sheets of nori.
11. Serve immediately with the pickled ginger, soy sauce, and wasabi, if using.

Prep tip: Don't want to bother with the rolling? Create a sushi bowl. Simply put brown rice in a bowl and top with the other ingredients.

PER SERVING (1 SUSHI ROLL): Calories: 261; Total fat: 8g; Total carbohydrates: 39g; Fiber: 5g; Protein: 10g; Sodium: 236mg

Chicken Salad Sandwich with Apples, Grapes, and Walnuts

GLUTEN-FREE (OPTION), MAKE AHEAD

MAKES 1 SANDWICH / TOTAL TIME: 10 MINUTES

In this recipe, chicken is combined with sweetness from grapes and apple and crunch from celery and walnuts, thus transforming bland chicken into a delicious sandwich. It's an example of synergy, when the whole is greater than the sum of its parts. To speed up your meal prep, double this recipe for two days' worth of sandwiches. Looking for a lighter lunch option? Omit the bread and serve it salad-style on extra Bibb lettuce.

2 tablespoons mayonnaise

1 teaspoon apple cider vinegar

⅛ teaspoon salt

¼ teaspoon ground black pepper

1 chicken breast, shredded

4 red seedless grapes, quartered

¼ apple, cored, peeled, and finely diced

½ celery stalk, finely chopped

1 tablespoon walnut pieces

2 slices whole grain bread (or gluten-free, if desired)

2 leaves Bibb lettuce

1. In a medium bowl, combine the mayonnaise, vinegar, salt, and pepper. Whisk to combine.

2. Add the chicken, grapes, apple, celery, and walnuts. Stir gently to combine.

3. Assemble the sandwich using the bread, chicken salad mixture, and lettuce.

Ingredient tip: This is an excellent recipe for leftovers from Lemon-Garlic Roast Chicken (page 91).

PER SERVING: Calories: 603; Total fat: 31g; Total carbohydrates: 56g; Fiber: 12g; Protein: 37g; Sodium: 968mg

IF YOU HAVE TO BUY LUNCH

Hey, no one's perfect. Sometimes, despite our best efforts, we fail to pack a lunch. There are also business lunches, where eating at a restaurant is a must. Here's what to do if you have to buy lunch.

- **Fill up on protein and veggies.** Large quantities of refined grains such as white bread and white rice will cause a spike in your blood sugar that can trigger sugar cravings later in the day. Considering real whole grains are few and far between when eating out, the best strategy is to focus on protein and veggies, thus limiting the amount of refined grains.

- **Make half of your plate veggies.** To achieve this, you will likely have to ask for extra vegetables. Or choose salad instead of fries. Not a fan of salads? You can often order a side of cooked veggies as a side for a burger or sandwich instead of the fries or salad.

- **Dress yourself.** Most restaurant salad dressings are loaded with sugar. Ask for oil and vinegar instead of salad dressing.

- **No nuts.** Candied nuts, as the name suggests, are coated in sugar. Watch out for them on salad.

- **Careful with condiments.** Ketchup contains free sugar. So do many other condiments. Stick with mustard and mayonnaise on a burger.

- **Avoid glaze.** It's a fancy word meaning coated in sugar. Stay away from glazed salmon, glazed chicken, glazed carrots, and the like. Barbeque sauce, too.

A Better Turkey Sandwich

GLUTEN-FREE (OPTION), MAKE AHEAD

MAKES 1 SANDWICH / PREP TIME: 5 MINUTES / TOTAL TIME: 15 MINUTES

This sandwich is inspired by a classic turkey club sandwich. However, I've removed the third piece of bread (which is too much starch for most people) and replaced it with a roasted red pepper. I'm always looking for delicious ways to eat more veggies. Roasted red peppers, sometimes called pimento, are available in jars in most supermarkets, especially those with a good Italian food or Mediterranean food section.

2 slices bacon

2 pieces whole grain bread (gluten-free, if desired)

1 roasted red pepper

2 pieces sliced turkey breast

1 tomato, sliced

1 leaf romaine lettuce

Mayonnaise

Dijon mustard

1. Lay the bacon slices in a cold skillet.
2. Over low-medium heat, cook the bacon. When the bacon starts to buckle and curl, use tongs to loosen the strips and flip them to cook on the other side. Keep flipping and turning the bacon so that it browns evenly.
3. When the bacon is cooked, remove the bacon from the skillet and put it on a paper towel–lined plate.
4. Toast the bread, if desired.
5. Slice the red pepper so it will lie flat. Pat it dry on a paper towel.
6. Assemble the sandwich using all of the ingredients as desired.

Prep tip: Cook extra bacon for use in future sandwiches or other dishes. For example, Classic Cobb Salad (page 49).

PER SERVING: Calories: 443; Total fat: 11g; Total carbohydrates: 56g; Fiber: 13g; Protein: 38g; Sodium: 1,198mg

Collard Green Wrap with Roast Beef and Quinoa

GLUTEN-FREE, MAKE AHEAD

MAKES 2 WRAPS / TOTAL TIME: 5 MINUTES

Swap out the tortillas for collard greens and get your carbohydrates from whole grain quinoa in this wrap. It took a while for me to figure out how to get collards to actually roll up. Once I figured out the shaved middle rib technique, I felt like shouting EUREKA! While this wrap uses simple ingredients, it's a whole new take on roast beef. When you cook quinoa for dinner one evening, make extra to use in these wraps.

2 collard leaves

4 slices roast beef

Dijon mustard

Mayonnaise

1 cup cooked quinoa

4 sun-dried tomatoes,

packed in oil

1. Shave the thickness off the middle rib of the collard greens so that you can roll each leaf from top to bottom.
2. Starting at the top of one leaf, place two pieces of roast beef. Spread with mustard and mayonnaise.
3. Place ½ cup quinoa on top of the roast beef in a line, perpendicular to the middle rib.
4. Pat the oil off of the tomatoes. Place 2 sun-dried tomatoes per wrap on top of the quinoa.
5. Tuck up one edge of the collard green as you would for a burrito. Starting at the top of the leaf, roll up the collard green.

Ingredient tip: Raw collard greens don't have the bitter flavor profile of many cooked leafy greens. As a result, this is a good recipe for those who want to get health benefits of leafy greens but don't like the taste of them cooked.

PER SERVING (1 WRAP): Calories: 233; Total fat: 6g; Total carbohydrates: 35g; Fiber: 5g; Protein: 12g; Sodium: 288mg

Southwest Steak Wrap

GLUTEN-FREE (OPTION), MAKE AHEAD

MAKES 1 WRAP / TOTAL TIME: 10 MINUTES

There's a reason black beans, corn, bell peppers, onion, and avocado are a classic combination. They taste great together! The natural sweetness of the corn and bell pepper play off the creaminess of the avocado. All work in harmony to set off the earthiness of the steak in this recipe. Here, I include them to provide a nutrient- and fiber-packed addition to this steak wrap.

¼ cup kernel corn, fresh, frozen, or canned

¼ cup black beans

1 tablespoon mayonnaise

1 teaspoon lime juice

Dash hot sauce, such as Tabasco

1 whole wheat tortilla (gluten-free wrap, if desired)

3 ounces cooked sirloin steak, sliced

2 leaves romaine lettuce

¼ red bell pepper, cut into strips

2 thin slices red onion

¼ avocado, sliced (optional)

1. Thoroughly drain and rinse the corn and beans.
2. In a small bowl, combine the mayonnaise, lime juice, and hot sauce.
3. Assemble the wrap. Add the lime-mayonnaise mixture as the last step before rolling.

Ingredient tip: Looking for directions on cooking your steak? Check out the Pan-Seared Steak with Carrot-Parsnip Mash recipe on page 108.

PER SERVING: Calories: 535; Total fat: 28g; Total carbohydrates: 45g; Fiber: 9g; Protein: 28g; Sodium: 463mg

5

SNACKS

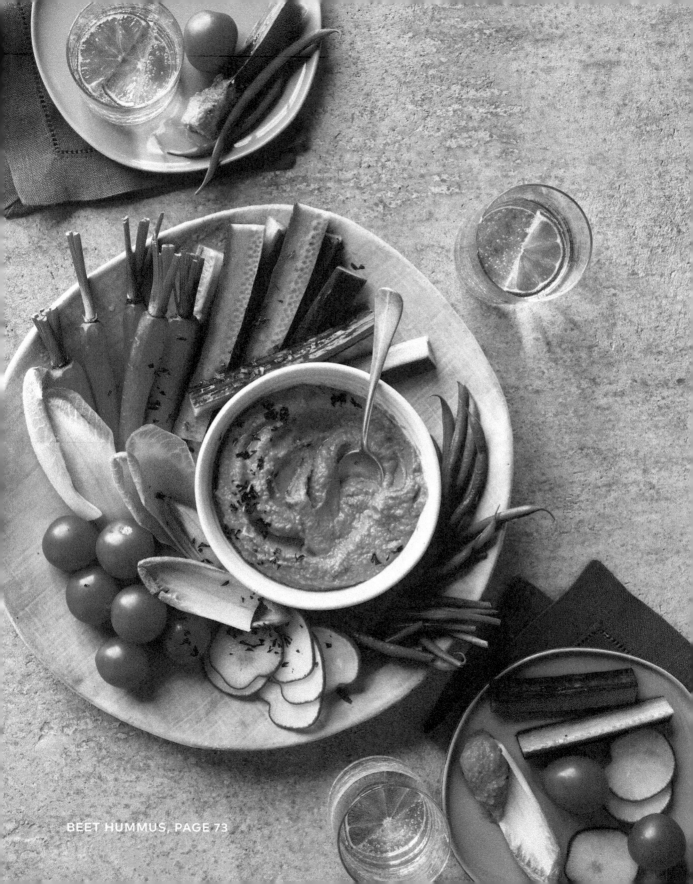

BEET HUMMUS, PAGE 73

Baba Ghanoush

VEGETARIAN, VEGAN, GLUTEN-FREE, MAKES GREAT LEFTOVERS

SERVES 4 / PREP TIME: 10 MINUTES / COOK TIME: 45 MINUTES TO 1 HOUR

While it has a fancy-sounding name, baba ghanoush is actually very easy to make. There are as many different ways to spell this traditional dip from the Mediterranean region as there are different ways to make it. As you know, I like things to be super simple. So, here's my simple recipe. Look for the rounder Mediterranean-style eggplant for this dish, not the long, skinny Asian eggplant. Here's a meal prep hack: Both the eggplant and garlic are flexible when it comes to oven temperature. I often add the eggplant and garlic to the oven when I'm cooking another dish.

1 eggplant

3 tablespoons plus 1 teaspoon extra-virgin olive oil, divided

1 head garlic

3 tablespoons lemon juice

⅛ teaspoon salt

1. Preheat the oven to 375°F.
2. Cut any loose, leafy parts off the eggplant. Pierce the skin with a fork, making pierce marks about 1 or 2 inches apart. Rub the eggplant with ½ teaspoon of the olive oil and put it in a metal or ceramic baking dish.
3. Remove the outermost skin of the garlic head (the loose stuff). Cut off the very top of the head, so the tip of each clove is exposed. Rub the entire head with ½ teaspoon of olive oil and wrap it in foil, shiny side inward. Put the package in the baking dish, alongside the eggplant.
4. Bake in the oven until the garlic is soft and fragrant and the eggplant is wrinkled and soft to the touch, about 45 minutes to 1 hour. Set aside and allow to cool.
5. Once cooled, remove half of the garlic cloves from the head and put them in a medium-size bowl or the bowl of a blender or food processor. Add the lemon juice, remaining olive oil, and salt.
6. Cut the eggplant in half lengthwise. With a spoon, scoop out the flesh. Add it to the mixture.

7. Blend the mixture until smooth. Adjust the ingredients to suit your taste and texture preferences (e.g., add the rest of the roasted garlic cloves if you want a more garlicky dip).

Ingredient tip: Leftover roasted garlic cloves taste fantastic on their own smashed onto a piece of crusty whole grain bread or a whole grain cracker.

PER SERVING: Calories: 146; Total fat: 12g; Total carbohydrates: 11g; Fiber: 4g; Protein: 2g; Sodium: 78mg

Carrot Yogurt Dip

VEGETARIAN, GLUTEN-FREE

SERVES 4 / PREP TIME: 5 MINUTES / TOTAL TIME: 20 MINUTES

Something magical happens in this recipe. It's an absolute crowd-pleaser whenever I bring it to a potluck, but no one ever believes me about how few ingredients are involved. So I'm sharing it with you here to prove that I'm not a liar! The slow, low cooking of the carrots causes their natural sugars to caramelize to delicious effect. Patience is your friend here. Keep stirring and waiting for the color change. That's your signal that the magic has occurred.

2 tablespoons extra-virgin olive oil

1½ cups grated carrots

1 cup plain, unsweetened Greek yogurt

¼ teaspoon ground black pepper

⅛ teaspoon salt

1. Warm the oil in a skillet over low-medium heat. Add the carrot. Cook, stirring frequently until the carrots are lightly browned and very soft, about 15 minutes.
2. Transfer the carrots to a serving bowl or storage container and allow to cool. Stir in the yogurt, pepper, and salt.

Storage tip: This recipe doesn't freeze well. Be sure to store leftovers in the refrigerator for 3 or 4 days maximum.

PER SERVING: Calories: 119; Total fat: 8g; Total carbohydrates: 6g; Fiber: 1g; Protein: 6g; Sodium: 127mg

Minted Pea Dip

VEGETARIAN, VEGAN, GLUTEN-FREE, MAKES GREAT LEFTOVERS

SERVES 2 / TOTAL TIME: 15 MINUTES

This bright, refreshing dip delivers more protein than you likely imagine. While most of us think of peas as vegetables, they are related to beans, lentils, and soy. As such, they contain some protein (4 grams in a ½-cup serving) and some iron too (1.3 grams in a ½-cup serving).

3 cups water

1 cup frozen peas

2 tablespoons fresh mint

1 tablespoon extra-virgin olive oil

1 tablespoon lemon juice

⅛ teaspoon salt

⅛ teaspoon ground black pepper

1. Bring the water to a boil in a medium saucepan. Add the peas. Cook for 1 minute. Drain into a colander and then transfer the peas to a bowl of cold water to stop the cooking.

2. In a blender, combine the peas and all the remaining ingredients. Purée until smooth.

Ingredient tip: This recipe is even better in the summer when fresh peas are in season.

PER SERVING: Calories: 116; Total fat: 7g; Total carbohydrates: 10g; Fiber: 3g; Protein: 4g; Sodium: 226mg

DIPPING YOUR WAY TO HEALTHY EATING

Dips get a bad rap. They're labeled unhealthy, and many people consider them kid food.

The kids have it right—dips are fun and delicious. Because dipping is fun and delicious, dips can be a great way to prevent you from being tempted by sugary snack foods. They can also help you eat your veggies. There's nothing wrong with some salad dressing (without free sugar) to go along with your baby carrots.

But don't stop your use of dips at salad dressing. Dips can also be nutrition powerhouses in and of themselves, containing veggies or protein-rich foods like beans. That's why this chapter contains so many recipes for dips. Use them to help fuel your sugar-free lifestyle.

White Bean Dip

VEGETARIAN, VEGAN, GLUTEN-FREE, MAKES GREAT LEFTOVERS

SERVES 4 / PREP TIME: 10 MINUTES / COOK TIME: 45 MINUTES

This white bean dip is super easy to make. Adjust the amounts of garlic, lemon juice, and olive oil to match your taste buds. You can use any white bean in this recipe, such as cannellini beans, white kidney beans, or white navy beans. Roasting garlic changes and mellows its flavor, so don't be afraid of the whole head of garlic that is called for in this recipe. It's not a typo!

1 head garlic

¼ cup plus ½ teaspoon extra-virgin olive oil, divided

1 (15½-ounce) can white beans

¼ cup lemon juice

1. Preheat the oven to 400°F.
2. Remove the outermost skin of the garlic head (the loose stuff). Cut off the very top of the head, so the tip of each clove is exposed. Rub the entire head with ½ teaspoon of olive oil and wrap it in foil, shiny side inward. Put it on a baking sheet or in a casserole dish.
3. Roast the garlic in the oven for about 45 minutes, or until the head gives off the distinct roasted garlic (not raw garlic) aroma and the cloves are squishy.
4. Allow to cool.
5. Drain and rinse the beans. Put the beans in a medium-size bowl.
6. To the beans, add half the olive oil, half of the lemon juice, and half of the cloves of garlic. Using a handheld blender, blend the mixture until it's smooth. Add more olive oil, lemon juice, and garlic to taste and to get the texture to the desired smoothness.

Ingredient tip: You can roast the garlic ahead of time to make this dip very quick to prepare.

PER SERVING: Calories: 220; Total fat: 15g; Total carbohydrates: 15g; Fiber: 5g; Protein: 5g; Sodium: 95mg

Black Bean Salsa

VEGETARIAN, VEGAN, GLUTEN-FREE, MAKES GREAT LEFTOVERS

SERVES 4 / TOTAL TIME: 10 MINUTES

Hey, we all like chips and salsa. Here, I up salsa's nutritional game by adding black beans for a healthy protein and fiber addition. The beans give this salsa more power to keep you full until dinner. Or, do like my friend Kim did. She's an exhausted new mom. When I gave her this recipe as I was testing it, she topped it with grilled chicken for an easy and delicious lunch.

1 (15½-ounce) can black beans

1 avocado, diced

1 red bell pepper, diced

½ cup white onion, diced

3 Roma tomatoes, diced

1 cup fresh cilantro, finely chopped

¼ cup fresh lime juice

¼ teaspoon salt

1. Drain and rinse the beans.
2. Add the remaining ingredients to a medium-size bowl or plastic storage container. Stir to combine.

Ingredient tip: Often, I'll use bottled lime juice in recipes. However, juice from fresh limes is really needed to make this recipe sing.

PER SERVING: Calories: 190; Total fat: 8g; Total carbohydrates: 26g; Fiber: 10g; Protein: 8g; Sodium: 246mg

Beet Hummus

VEGETARIAN, VEGAN, GLUTEN-FREE, MAKES GREAT LEFTOVERS

SERVES 4 / TOTAL TIME: 15 MINUTES

I'm all about creative and delicious recipes that provide ways to eat more veggies. Here, I've upgraded the usual hummus for one with beets. The result is a beautiful pink color. It's a hit with adults who aren't crazy about beets, and its pink color is also a hit with picky eater little princes and princesses. You can also use it instead of the regular hummus in Toasted Hummus Garden Sandwiches (page 52).

1 (15½-ounce) can chickpeas

1 cup canned, sliced beets

¼ cup extra-virgin olive oil

¼ cup lemon juice (fresh or bottled)

¼ cup tahini (sesame seed butter)

1 garlic clove, minced

¼ teaspoon salt

Combine all of the ingredients in a blender. Purée until smooth.

Storage tip: Hummus doesn't freeze well—the texture just doesn't hold up. So be sure to eat up this recipe in the first 3 or 4 days after making it (that's how long it keeps well in the fridge).

PER SERVING: Calories: 332; Total fat: 23g; Total carbohydrates: 25g; Fiber: 7g; Protein: 9g; Sodium: 291mg

Savory Popcorn, Two Ways

VEGETARIAN, GLUTEN-FREE, MAKES GREAT LEFTOVERS

SERVES 2 / TOTAL TIME: 10 MINUTES

Popcorn gets a bad nutritional rap, but popcorn itself is a real whole food. It's the drowning of those whole grains in imitation "buttery" topping and pounds of salt or free sugar that is the problem. Instead, here are two healthier options for popcorn. The Parmesan and nutritional yeast provide the umami flavor that makes popcorn so irresistible. Nutritional yeast is a common ingredient in some styles of vegetarian cooking.

FOR THE POPCORN

1 teaspoon vegetable oil

¼ cup popping corn kernels

1 teaspoon butter

FOR THE ITALIAN STYLE

2 teaspoons grated

Parmesan cheese

1 teaspoon dried basil

1 teaspoon dried oregano

FOR THE WEST COAST STYLE

2 teaspoons nutritional yeast

1 teaspoon chili powder

¼ teaspoon salt

1. In a large saucepan over medium heat, combine the vegetable oil and popcorn. Shake to coat the kernels in oil. Cover the pot. Heat the popcorn, shaking frequently, until the popping sounds come to a stop.
2. In a small bowl, combine the seasonings. Mix well.
3. Add the butter to the popped popcorn in the hot saucepan and toss to coat.
4. Transfer the popcorn to a serving bowl. Toss with your choice of seasoning mixture.

Storage tip: Popcorn is a tasty snack served immediately, when it's still hot, or store it in a resealable storage container and serve it cold.

PER SERVING (ITALIAN): Calories: 129; Total fat: 6g; Total carbohydrates: 20g; Fiber: 4g; Protein: 4g; Sodium: 63mg

PER SERVING (WEST COAST): Calories: 124; Total fat: 5g; Total carbohydrates: 21g; Fiber: 4g; Protein: 4g; Sodium: 304mg

Chocolate Chia Pudding

VEGETARIAN, VEGAN, GLUTEN-FREE, MAKE AHEAD

SERVES 2 / TOTAL TIME: 35 MINUTES, PLUS OVERNIGHT TO SET

This delicious treat is actually good for you because it's made with chia seeds rich in protein, iron, and fiber. The result is a gel or pudding-like consistency, similar to tapioca pudding. I love the combination of orange and chocolate, so I will often add a drop or two of orange blossom water to the mixture before allowing it to set. You can find orange blossom water in any supermarket or specialty food store that carries Middle Eastern foods.

3 tablespoons chia seeds

1 cup milk (dairy, plant-based alternative, or even canned coconut milk)

1 tablespoon cocoa powder

1. Combine all of the ingredients in a container with a lid. Stir well to thoroughly combine.
2. Leave at room temperature for 30 minutes.
3. Refrigerate overnight.

Preparation tip: Don't be tempted to skip the step of leaving the pudding at room temperature before putting it in the refrigerator. Skipping this step may result in preventing the gel from forming.

PER SERVING: Calories: 146; Total fat: 6g; Total carbohydrates: 14g; Fiber: 8g; Protein: 9g; Sodium: 61mg

Roasted Chickpeas, Two Ways

VEGETARIAN, VEGAN, GLUTEN-FREE, MAKES GREAT LEFTOVERS

SERVES 4 / PREP TIME: 5 MINUTES / COOK TIME: 30 MINUTES

Chickpeas are high in vegan-source protein, high in fiber, a source of low-glycemic carbs, and contain lots of other nutrients. You likely know them as the main ingredient in hummus. Here, I share a different way to enjoy chickpeas as a snack: roasted. I'm including two seasoning mixtures that I enjoy for roasted chickpeas, but the flavor combinations are endless. Feel free to play with your seasonings. Definitely take the time to thoroughly dry your chickpeas. Otherwise, they will be mushy.

FOR THE BASE

1 (15½-ounce) can chickpeas

FOR THE SAVORY ROASTED STYLE

2 tablespoons extra-virgin olive oil

½ teaspoon garlic powder

½ teaspoon ground cumin

¼ teaspoon salt

¼ teaspoon ground black pepper

FOR THE GARAM MASALA STYLE

2 tablespoons extra-virgin olive oil

1 teaspoon garam masala

¼ teaspoon salt

1. Preheat the oven to 400°F.
2. Drain and rinse the chickpeas. Pat them dry.
3. Combine all the other ingredients in a medium-size bowl.
4. Toss the chickpeas in the mixture, coating the chickpeas well.
5. Line a baking sheet with parchment paper. Spread the coated chickpeas onto the parchment paper-lined sheet in a single layer.
6. Bake the chickpeas in the oven for 30 minutes, stirring every 10 minutes.

Baking tip: Keep a close eye on your chickpeas while they bake. You're looking for them to turn a golden brown color. When you taste them, they should have a crunchy shell and be soft in the middle.

PER SERVING: Calories: 161; Total fat: 9g; Total carbohydrates: 17g; Fiber: 5g; Protein: 5g; Sodium: 149mg

Spiced Nuts

VEGETARIAN, VEGAN, GLUTEN-FREE (OPTION), MAKES GREAT LEFTOVERS

SERVES 8 / TOTAL TIME: 5 MINUTES

Your home will smell amazing when you make this spiced nut recipe. Toasting nuts brings out their natural flavors. Here, they're paired with an alluring mixture of spices to make for a crave-worthy snack. You can mix and match the nuts in this recipe—use all almonds or double up the cashews and omit the pecans. Walnuts and hazelnuts would also work well here.

1 teaspoon salt

½ teaspoon pepper

1 teaspoon cinnamon

½ teaspoon curry powder

¼ teaspoon cloves

¼ teaspoon cumin

1 cup almonds

½ cup cashews

½ cup pecans

1 tablespoon reduced-sodium soy sauce (or gluten-free tamari, if desired)

1. Combine the spices in a small bowl.
2. In a skillet over medium heat, add the nuts and spices. Cook, stirring constantly, for 2 minutes, or until the mixture is fragrant.
3. Add in the soy sauce. Stir for 30 seconds.
4. Remove from the heat.

Storage tip: Serve the nuts warm or allow them to cool and store them in a resealable storage container.

PER SERVING: Calories: 201; Total fat: 18g; Total carbohydrates: 8g; Fiber: 3g; Protein: 6g; Sodium: 364mg

Lentil-Coconut Energy Bites

VEGAN, VEGETARIAN, GLUTEN-FREE, MAKES GREAT LEFTOVERS

SERVES 5 / TOTAL TIME: 15 MINUTES

These energy bites are a fantastic way to get acquainted with lentils. Lentils are the easiest to digest of all beans and pulses. These bites are a great no free sugar alternative to sugary granola bars. With their protein, fiber, and low-glycemic index carbohydrates, these bites will keep you full, thus preventing you from being tempted by sugary snacks.

½ cup pumpkin seeds

4 dates

⅓ cup rolled oats

½ teaspoon ground cinnamon

½ teaspoon vanilla extract

½ cup lentils (canned or cooked from dry)

¼ cup unsweetened, medium-size shredded coconut

1. In a blender or food processor, purée the pumpkin seeds until smooth. Add the dates and continue to purée.
2. Once you reach a paste-like consistency, add in the oats, cinnamon, vanilla, and lentils.
3. Transfer the mixture to a bowl.
4. Using your hands, roll the mixture into about 10 small balls.
5. Lay a piece of parchment paper on a flat work surface. Sprinkle with the shredded coconut. Roll the lentil bites in the coconut.

Storage tip: These need to be kept refrigerated. Store them in the refrigerator for 3 or 4 days, or freeze part of your batch in a resealable plastic storage bag for 2 or 3 months.

PER SERVING: Calories: 117; Total fat: 4g; Total carbohydrates: 17g; Fiber: 3g; Protein: 4g; Sodium: 3mg

Apple-Cinnamon Muffins

VEGETARIAN, GLUTEN-FREE (OPTION), MAKES GREAT LEFTOVERS

MAKES 12 MUFFINS / PREP TIME: 10 MINUTES / COOK TIME: 20 TO 25 MINUTES

While I love to cook, I'm not a baker. So you know that if I'm sharing a baking recipe, it must be really easy and foolproof. In this recipe, the sweetness comes from the applesauce and puréed raisins. You'll never believe that there isn't any free sugar. If you are baking-inclined, feel free to play with this recipe. The puréed raisin hack works well for all sorts of muffins.

Cooking oil spray

¼ cup boiling water

½ cup raisins

2½ cups whole wheat flour (or gluten-free flour, if desired)

1 teaspoon baking soda

½ teaspoon salt

1 tablespoon cinnamon

3 tablespoons vegetable oil

2 teaspoons white vinegar

½ cup unsweetened applesauce

¾ cup milk

½ cup walnuts

1. Preheat the oven to 350°F.
2. Spray the muffin tin with cooking oil spray.
3. Boil the water (a kettle works well). Add the raisins and water to a blender. Soak the raisins in the boiling water for 5 minutes, then purée.
4. In a large bowl, stir together the flour, baking soda, salt, and cinnamon.
5. In a medium bowl, beat together the oil, vinegar, applesauce, and milk.
6. Add the wet ingredients to the dry ingredients. Add in the raisin mixture and walnuts. Mix just until combined (do not overmix). Divide the batter evenly among the 12 muffin cups.
7. Bake for 20 to 25 minutes.

Storage tip: These muffins freeze well. Put them in a resealable plastic storage bag.

PER SERVING (1 Muffin): Calories: 177; Total fat: 7g; Total carbohydrates: 26g; Fiber: 4g; Protein: 5g; Sodium: 210mg

Fruit and Nut Squares

VEGETARIAN, VEGAN, GLUTEN-FREE, MAKES GREAT LEFTOVERS

MAKES 24 SQUARES / PREP TIME: 10 MINUTES / COOK TIME: 15 MINUTES

If date squares and granola bars had a baby, it would look (and taste) like this. These filling squares are naturally sweet from all the dried fruit that they contain. When making the recipe, take the time to dice your fruit into really small pieces. If you leave your fruit pieces too large, the bars may crumble apart.

3 tablespoons ground flaxseed

½ cup water

1 cup goji berries

1½ cups dried apricots, finely diced

1 cup dates, pitted and finely diced

1 cup brown rice flour

1 cup sunflower seeds

1 cup pecans, chopped

1 cup rolled oats (gluten-free, if desired)

½ cup applesauce

2 teaspoons vanilla

1. In a small bowl, combine the flaxseed with water and set aside.
2. Preheat the oven to 350°F.
3. Line 9-by-13-inch pan with parchment paper.
4. In a large bowl, toss the goji berries, apricots, and dates in the flour to coat.
5. Add the sunflower seeds, pecans, oats, applesauce, vanilla, and flaxseed mixture.
6. Transfer the mixture to the pan. Press firmly to create an even thickness.
7. Bake for 12 minutes.
8. Allow the squares to cool before removing them from the pan and cutting them into bars.

Storage tip: These bars freeze well. Put them in a resealable plastic bag.

PER SERVING (1 Square): Calories: 165; Total fat: 7g; Total carbohydrates: 25g; Fiber: 4g; Protein: 4g; Sodium: 2mg

Deviled-Style Guacamole Eggs

VEGETARIAN, GLUTEN-FREE, MAKE AHEAD, MAKES GREAT LEFTOVERS

SERVES 3 / TOTAL TIME: 10 MINUTES

Isn't it amazing how food can connect us with memories? I love deviled eggs. They remind me of my Grannie, who used to make them for me from early childhood, right up until my twenties. Here, I combine them with another lifelong snack favorite, guacamole. My Grannie absolutely adored avocados, so I think that she would wholeheartedly approve of this snack mash-up.

1 avocado

1 Roma tomato

2 tablespoons cilantro, finely chopped

1 garlic clove, minced

1 teaspoon lime juice

Pinch salt

⅛ teaspoon ground black pepper

6 hard-boiled eggs

1. Remove the avocado flesh from the peel and pit. Dice the avocado flesh and the tomato.
2. In a medium-size bowl, combine the avocado, tomato, cilantro, garlic, lime juice, cilantro, salt, and pepper. Mash everything together with a fork.
3. Peel and cut the hard-boiled eggs in half. Scoop out the yolks. Mix the yolks into the avocado mixture.
4. Fill the hollow in your egg whites with the guacamole mixture.

Storage tip: If you are planning to make this snack ahead of time, prepare the guacamole but do not prepare the eggs. Store the guacamole in an airtight container in the refrigerator. When you are ready to serve the snack, prepare steps 3 and 4.

PER SERVING: Calories: 273; Total fat: 20g; Total carbohydrates: 10g; Fiber: 5g; Protein: 15g; Sodium: 182mg

Avocado Halves with Shrimp

GLUTEN-FREE, MAKES GREAT LEFTOVERS

SERVES 2 / TOTAL TIME: 5 MINUTES

These snacks are as easy as they are elegant. It's amazing how so few ingredients can work together so synergistically. Did you know that avocados are not only a source of healthy fat but also a good source of fiber? Combined with the protein in the shrimp, this snack will keep you satisfied for hours.

1 avocado

1 (4-ounce) can baby shrimp

½ teaspoon balsamic vinegar

Pinch salt

1. Cut the avocado in half and remove the pit.
2. Rinse the shrimp. Put a scoop of shrimp in the hollow made by the avocado pit.
3. Sprinkle with the balsamic vinegar and salt.

Ingredient tip: Substitute the canned baby shrimp with leftover cooked shrimp, such as those in Lemon-Garlic Shrimp Kebabs (page 118).

PER SERVING: Calories: 204; Total fat: 14g; Total carbohydrates: 7g; Fiber: 6g; Protein: 16g; Sodium: 174mg

6

POULTRY & MEAT

PINEAPPLE-PORK KEBABS, PAGE 97

Chicken Soup with Quinoa

GLUTEN-FREE, MAKE AHEAD, MAKES GREAT LEFTOVERS

SERVES 4 / PREP TIME: 10 MINUTES / COOK TIME: 20 MINUTES

I believe that everyone needs a chicken soup recipe in their repertoire. Okay, every nonvegetarian, that is. Homemade soup is the perfect way to use up leftovers from a roast chicken. I like this recipe in particular, because it's like two soups in one. When eaten immediately after cooking, it's a broth soup. However, the quinoa continues to expand, so leftovers are thick, like a stew.

1 tablespoon extra-virgin olive oil

½ cup yellow onion, diced

1 cup celery, diced

2 cups carrots, diced

2 garlic cloves, minced

2 quarts (8 cups) chicken stock, vegetable stock, or water

1 cup quinoa

1 bay leaf

1 teaspoon dried thyme

⅛ teaspoon salt

1 teaspoon ground black pepper

Meat from 4 pieces of chicken (such as 2 breasts, 2 thighs)

1. Heat the oil in a large saucepan over medium heat. Add the onion, celery, carrots, and garlic. Sauté until the onion is translucent, 3 or 4 minutes.

2. Add the stock, quinoa, bay leaf, thyme, salt, and pepper. Cover, increase the heat to maximum, and bring to a boil. Lower to low-medium heat and simmer for 10 minutes, stirring frequently. Add the chicken in the final 2 minutes of cooking. If the soup gets too thick, add more stock. To serve, divide into 4 serving bowls.

Ingredient tip: This is a fantastic recipe for leftovers from roasting a whole chicken, such as from Lemon-Garlic Roast Chicken (page 91), or leftovers from a store-bought whole roast chicken.

PER SERVING: Calories: 371; Total fat: 11g; Total carbohydrates: 38g; Fiber: 6g; Protein: 31g; Sodium: 1,204mg

HOW LONG DO THOSE LEFTOVERS KEEP?

After doing the meal prep work of cooking leftovers, you want to make sure that you eat the food before it goes bad. Here are the FDA's guidelines for how long to keep food to minimize the risk of foodborne illness (what we commonly call food poisoning).

Food	Refrigerator	Freezer
Soups and stews (vegetarian or containing meat or poultry)	3 to 4 days	2 to 3 months
Raw hamburger	1 to 2 days	3 to 4 months
Raw steak	3 to 5 days	6 to 12 months
Cooked meat	3 to 4 days	2 to 3 months
Raw pork chops	3 to 5 days	4 to 6 months
Cooked ham	3 to 4 days	1 to 2 months
Raw chicken	1 to 2 days	9 months
Raw ground turkey	1 to 2 days	3 to 4 months
Cooked chicken, plain	3 to 4 days	4 months
Cooked chicken in sauce	3 to 4 days	6 months
Raw lean fish	1 to 2 days	6 to 8 months
Raw fatty fish	1 to 2 days	2 to 3 months
Raw shrimp and other shellfish	1 to 2 days	3 to 6 months
Cooked fish	3 to 4 days	4 to 6 months
Canned seafood, after opening	3 to 4 days	2 months
Eggs, (raw, in shell)	3 to 5 weeks	Don't freeze
Hard-boiled eggs	1 week	Don't freeze

Chicken and Grape Kebabs

GLUTEN-FREE, MAKE AHEAD

SERVES 4 / PREP TIME: 15 MINUTES / COOK TIME: 15 MINUTES, PLUS 4 HOURS TO OVERNIGHT

The zing of the lemon-garlic chicken and the sweetness of the red bell pepper and grapes harmonize together in this dish. I chose green grapes and red pepper because I found that color combination to be the most appealing.

2 tablespoons extra-virgin olive oil

1 lemon zest

2 tablespoons lemon juice

2 garlic cloves, minced

1 teaspoon ground cumin

½ teaspoon ground coriander

1 teaspoon oregano

½ teaspoon salt

2 pounds boneless, skinless chicken breast

8 skewers, metal or wooden

2 red bell peppers

1½ cups seedless green grapes

Cooking oil spray

1. In a medium bowl, combine the olive oil, lemon zest, lemon juice, garlic, cumin, coriander, oregano, and salt.
2. Cut the chicken breast into ¾-inch cubes. Add it to the marinade and toss to coat. Cover and refrigerate for 4 hours or overnight.
3. If using wooden skewers, put them in a large shallow dish and soak them in water while you prepare the remaining ingredients.
4. Cut the bell pepper into ¾-inch pieces. Create a production line with the chicken, grapes, and bell pepper. Thread the ingredients onto the skewers, alternating among the ingredients.
5. For the oven: Preheat the oven to 400°F. Spray a baking sheet with cooking oil spray. Place the skewers on the pan and cook for 15 minutes, or until the chicken is cooked.
6. For the grill: Heat the grill on medium heat. Spray the grill with cooking oil spray. Grill, turning frequently, for 13 minutes, or until the chicken is cooked.
7. Serve while still on the skewers (my preference) or remove the chicken, peppers, and grapes from the skewers before plating.

PER SERVING: Calories: 329; Total fat: 12g; Total carbohydrates: 12g; Fiber: 2g; Protein: 47g; Sodium: 653mg

Chicken and Snap Peas Stir-Fry

GLUTEN-FREE (OPTION), MAKE AHEAD

SERVES 4 / PREP TIME: 10 MINUTES / COOK TIME: 10 MINUTES

Crisp snap peas and crunchy water chestnuts combine with chicken and refreshing ginger in this satisfying stir-fry. I kept it simple here, but you can always up your vegetable game by adding some Asian greens (e.g., bok choy) and bean sprouts. That's the beauty of stir-fry—it's endlessly adaptable.

2 teaspoons cornstarch

2 tablespoons plus 2 teaspoons vegetable oil, divided

2 teaspoons sesame oil

2 tablespoons reduced-sodium soy sauce, divided (or gluten-free tamari, if desired)

2 tablespoons rice vinegar (unseasoned)

½ teaspoon ground black pepper

¼ teaspoon red pepper flakes (optional)

4 boneless, skinless chicken breasts

8 cups snap peas or snow peas

1 (8-ounce) can water chestnuts, drained

6 scallions, sliced

2 garlic cloves, minced

1-by-1-inch piece ginger, minced

4 cups cooked brown rice

4 tablespoons sesame seeds

1. In a medium-size bowl, combine the cornstarch, 2 teaspoons vegetable oil, sesame oil, soy sauce, rice vinegar, black pepper, and red pepper flakes, if using. Set aside.
2. Cut the chicken into bite-size pieces.
3. Heat the 2 tablespoons of vegetable oil in a large skillet over medium heat. Add the chicken and let cook for 1 minute without moving. Then turn the chicken over and add the peas, water chestnuts, scallions, garlic, and ginger. Sauté, stirring constantly, for 2 minutes.
4. Stir the sauce to combine it and then add it to the skillet. Sauté, stirring constantly, for 5 minutes, until the sauce thickens and chicken is cooked through.
5. Serve over the brown rice and garnish with the sesame seeds. Serve with extra soy sauce, if desired.

Equipment tip: A wok, if you have one, is ideal for this recipe as it allows the veggies to get even heat, resulting in tender-crisp veggies.

PER SERVING: Calories: 572; Total fat: 21g; Total carbohydrates: 65g; Fiber: 9g; Protein: 34g; Sodium: 479mg

Chicken Tacos

GLUTEN-FREE

SERVES 4 / PREP TIME: 10 MINUTES / COOK TIME: 5 MINUTES

Taco Tuesdays, here you come! In only 15 minutes, you can have this delicious dinner, made from scratch. I've created this recipe to be veggie-heavy with four full bell peppers. As a dietitian, I can't help squeezing in extra veggies. If you find it to be too much, use only one bell pepper. Mix and match your favorite garnishes to create tacos in your own unique style.

2 teaspoons chili powder

2 teaspoons cumin

1 teaspoon garlic powder

¼ teaspoon salt

¼ teaspoon ground black pepper

½ teaspoon paprika

¼ teaspoon cayenne

2 tablespoons lime juice

4 boneless, skinless chicken breasts

2 green bell peppers

2 red bell peppers

1 tablespoon vegetable oil

8 corn taco shells

1 avocado, sliced, for garnish (optional)

1 jar salsa, no added sugar, for garnish (optional)

Sour cream or plain yogurt, for garnish (optional)

Hot sauce, for garnish (optional)

24 sprigs cilantro, for garnish (optional)

1 lime, quartered, for garnish (optional)

1. In a small bowl, combine the spices with the lime juice. Stir to combine.
2. Thinly slice the chicken breasts. Dredge the chicken in the spice mixture.
3. Thinly slice the bell peppers.
4. Heat the oil in a large skillet over medium heat. Add the bell pepper and chicken.
5. Sauté 3 to 5 minutes, until the chicken is cooked through.
6. Assemble your tacos in corn taco shells, garnished with the optional ingredients as desired.

Ingredient tip: This recipe also works well with leftover roast chicken. Toss the chicken in the spice mixture and add to the skillet for the final minute of cooking the bell peppers to heat the chicken.

PER SERVING: Calories: 272; Total fat: 11g; Total carbohydrates: 20g; Fiber: 4g; Protein: 25g; Sodium: 342mg

Lemon-Garlic Roast Chicken

GLUTEN-FREE, MAKES GREAT LEFTOVERS

SERVES 4 / PREP TIME: 10 MINUTES / COOK TIME: 45 MINUTES

This recipe is super simple. Yet it creates a sophisticated-tasting chicken that will impress dinner guests. Cook it on a lazy Sunday and you'll have leftovers for recipes like Classic Cobb Salad (page 49) and Chicken Tacos (page 90). This recipe uses a whole bird that is already cut into the individual pieces. Look for it in your local supermarket.

4 tablespoons extra-virgin olive oil, divided

1 (3 to 4 pound) chicken, cut into 8 parts (2 breasts, 2 thighs, 2 legs, 2 wings)

1 head garlic

1 lemon

1 teaspoon dried rosemary

½ teaspoon salt

½ teaspoon ground black pepper

1. Preheat the oven to 400°F.
2. Spread 1 tablespoon of the oil on the bottom of a 9¼-by-13¼-inch (3 quart) glass lasagna pan.
3. Pat the chicken pieces dry with a paper towel. Arrange the chicken pieces in the pan so that all the pieces are skin-side up.
4. Remove the outermost skin (the loose stuff) from the garlic head. Break the garlic head into individual cloves, but keep the cloves whole. Scatter the whole garlic cloves around the pan.
5. Zest the lemon, then cut it in half. Nestle the two half lemons, cut-side up, in the dish, in the spaces between the chicken pieces.
6. Sprinkle the rosemary over the dish.
7. Divide the lemon zest, salt, and pepper over chicken pieces. Pour 3 tablespoons of the oil over top of the chicken pieces.
8. Bake in the oven for 30 minutes. Then lower the heat to 350°F and bake for an additional 15 minutes, or until the internal temperature of the chicken breasts is 165°F and the temperature of the thighs is 170°F when tested with a meat thermometer.

Continued

9. To serve, allow people to choose their favorite parts, such as the breast, thigh, etc.

Storage tip: Store cooked chicken in the fridge for 3 or 4 days or in the freezer for up to 4 months.

PER SERVING: Calories: 327; Total fat: 22g; Total carbohydrates: 5g; Fiber: 1g; Protein: 30g; Sodium: 449mg

Chicken Cassoulet

GLUTEN-FREE, MAKES GREAT LEFTOVERS

SERVES 4 / PREP TIME: 10 MINUTES / COOK TIME: 45 MINUTES

There must be as many cassoulet recipes as there are French kitchens. It's a timeless (and delicious) dish. I've used chicken drumsticks, but you can also use chicken thighs or a combination of the two. Don't use chicken breast in this recipe because the meat is too dry. I'm a fan of recipes that introduce beans and lentils to nonvegetarians. Beans and lentils are high in fiber and contain low-glycemic index carbohydrates. As such, they provide steady energy without any blood sugar spikes.

1 tablespoon extra-virgin olive oil

6 chicken drumsticks

¾ pound kielbasa sausage, cut into ½-inch slices

1 yellow onion, diced

3 cups diced carrots

1 garlic clove

3 tablespoons tomato paste

2 bay leaves

2 (15½-ounce) cans cannellini beans (white navy or white northern beans work too), drained

1 cup white wine

1 cup water or chicken stock

1 teaspoon thyme

¼ teaspoon salt

½ teaspoon ground black pepper

1. Heat the oil over medium-high heat in a large nonstick saucepan with a lid. When the oil is hot, add the chicken and sausage. Turn the chicken occasionally to start browning it on all sides, 7 minutes total. Transfer the chicken and sausages to a plate.

2. Turn the heat down to medium, add the onion and carrots to the saucepan. Sauté, stirring frequently, until the onion starts to become translucent, about 4 minutes. Add the garlic and cook 30 seconds. Add the tomato paste and cook for 1 minute. Add the remaining ingredients. Cook for 30 minutes, stirring occasionally, until the wine has reduced and the chicken is cooked through. To serve, divide among 4 serving dishes.

Ingredient tip: Read the labels carefully on chicken stock. Surprisingly, most brands contain free sugar.

PER SERVING: Calories: 714; Total fat: 42g; Total carbohydrates: 50g; Fiber: 15g; Protein: 48g; Sodium: 1,870mg

Turkey-Stuffed Zucchini

GLUTEN-FREE

SERVES 4 / PREP TIME: 10 MINUTES / COOK TIME: 30 MINUTES

Ground turkey, known for being dry, is given a lot of moisture here from the tomato sauce and zucchini. Save the zucchini that you scoop out for use in a pasta. For example, it would be a delicious addition to Sausage and Pepper Pasta (page 103) or Beans and Greens Pesto Pasta (page 154). It will keep in the refrigerator for 3 or 4 days. Add brown rice to create a balanced meal.

2 medium zucchinis

1 tablespoon extra-virgin olive oil

½ cup finely diced onion

1 garlic clove, minced

1 pound ground turkey

⅛ teaspoon salt

½ teaspoon ground black pepper

1½ cups tomato sauce

2 teaspoons balsamic vinegar

1 teaspoon dried oregano

1 teaspoon dried basil

2 tablespoons grated Parmesan (optional)

1. Preheat the oven to 400°F.

2. Cut the ends off the zucchinis. Cut them in half longways (to create a boat that we'll stuff). Scoop out the seeds and some of the flesh, leaving ½-inch-thick zucchini walls and bottom. Place the zucchini in a metal baking dish, cavity-side up.

3. Heat the oil in a large skillet over low-medium heat. Sauté the onions until translucent, about 4 minutes. Add the diced garlic and sauté for 30 seconds.

4. Turn the heat up to medium. Add the turkey, salt, and pepper. Sauté for 1 minute.

5. Add the tomato sauce, vinegar, oregano, and basil. Sauté for 2 or 3 minutes.

6. Fill the zucchini boats with the turkey mixture and top with the Parmesan, if using.

7. Cover the pan with foil.

8. Bake for 20 minutes, until the zucchini is cooked. To serve, place one half zucchini on each plate.

Storage tip: This recipe makes great refrigerated leftovers, but it doesn't freeze well. Store your stuffed zucchinis in the refrigerator for 3 or 4 days.

PER SERVING: Calories: 237; Total fat: 12g; Total carbohydrates: 13g; Fiber: 3g; Protein: 25g; Sodium: 661mg

Split Pea Soup with Ham

GLUTEN-FREE, MAKE AHEAD, MAKES GREAT LEFTOVERS

SERVES 6 / PREP TIME: 10 MINUTES / COOK TIME: 65 MINUTES, PLUS SOAKING OVERNIGHT

This is a recipe to make on a cold, dark winter day when you want to cozy up in the house. This recipe evokes a canned soup that many Canadians, myself included, grew up eating. While this soup takes a long time to cook, there really isn't a lot of work involved in preparing it. You just need to be home long enough to stir it occasionally while it simmers away. And remember to soak the peas the night before.

2 cups split peas

1 tablespoon extra-virgin olive oil

2 cups diced carrots

2 cups diced celery

1 cup diced onion

1½ cups cooked ham, diced

8 cups vegetable stock, chicken stock, or water

1 bay leaf

2 teaspoon thyme

1 teaspoon salt

1 teaspoon ground black pepper

1 cup whole milk (1% or 2% milk also work, but you won't get as rich of a soup)

1. Put the peas in a medium-size bowl. Add enough water so that the water comes up 1½ inches above the peas. Soak overnight.
2. Heat the oil in a large stockpot over medium heat.
3. Add the carrots, celery, and onion. Sauté 4 or 5 minutes, until the onion is translucent.
4. Add the ham. Sauté for 1 minute.
5. Add the stock, peas, bay leaf, thyme, salt, and pepper and increase the heat to high. Cover and bring to a boil. Reduce the heat and simmer, stirring frequently for 1 hour, or until the peas are cooked.
6. Add the milk and simmer for 5 more minutes. Divide the soup among serving bowls and top with a dash of ground black pepper. (To make the soup dairy free, enjoy it immediately without adding the milk.)

Storage tip: This recipe makes a big batch of soup. Divide it up. Store the amount that you will eat in 3 or 4 days in the refrigerator. Store the remainder in the freezer for up to 2 or 3 months.

PER SERVING: Calories: 324; Total fat: 6g; Total carbohydrates: 52g; Fiber: 17g; Protein: 29g; Sodium: 1,959mg

Pineapple-Pork Kebabs

GLUTEN-FREE (OPTION), MAKE AHEAD

SERVES 4 / PREP TIME: 15 MINUTES / COOK TIME: 15 TO 20 MINUTES, PLUS 4 HOURS TO OVERNIGHT TO MARINATE

I love kebabs. They are such a summertime staple. However, I live in an apartment without a balcony, so I'm always looking for kebab recipes that can be cooked in the oven. This recipe works equally well in the oven as it does on the grill. The same is true for the Chicken and Grape Kebabs (page 88). Often grilled pork is covered in free sugar. Here, the pineapple and cherry tomatoes provide natural sweetness.

½ cup reduced-sodium soy sauce (or gluten-free tamari, if desired)

3 tablespoons extra-virgin olive oil

1 cup diced yellow onion

5 garlic cloves, minced

1 teaspoon ground black pepper

¼ teaspoon red pepper flakes

2 pounds boneless pork loin

8 skewers, metal or wooden

1 green bell pepper

1½ cups pineapple, cubed

1½ cups cherry tomatoes

Cooking oil spray

1. In a medium-size bowl, combine the soy sauce, olive oil, onion, garlic, black pepper, and red pepper flakes. Cut the pork into 1-inch cubes. Add the pork and toss to coat. Cover and refrigerate at least 4 hours to overnight.

2. If using wooden skewers, put them in a large shallow dish and soak them in water while you prepare the remaining ingredients.

3. Cut the bell pepper and pineapple into 1-inch pieces. Leave the cherry tomatoes whole.

4. Create a production line with your ingredients. Thread the ingredients onto the skewers, alternating among the ingredients.

5. For the oven: Preheat the oven to 400°F. Spray a baking sheet with cooking oil spray. Put the skewers on the pan and cook for 20 minutes, or until the pork is cooked.

6. For the grill: Heat the grill on medium heat. Spray the grill with cooking oil spray. Grill, turning frequently for 15 minutes, or until the pork is cooked.

Continued

7. Serve while still on the skewers (my preference) or remove the pork, peppers, tomatoes, and pineapple from the skewers before plating.

Ingredient tip: A whole pineapple creates much more than you'll need for this recipe. Your supermarket may sell pineapple already cut into cubes. Or buy a whole pineapple and enjoy the remaining pineapple in Halibut with Tropical Fruit Salsa (page 127).

PER SERVING: Calories: 507; Total fat: 27g; Total carbohydrates: 21g; Fiber: 3g; Protein: 46g; Sodium: 1,960mg

Pork Lettuce Wraps

GLUTEN-FREE (OPTION), MAKES GREAT LEFTOVERS

SERVES 4 / PREP TIME: 15 MINUTES / COOK TIME: 5 MINUTES

The refreshing vegetables and flavorful herbs in this recipe make it a delicious, light summertime meal. Are you easing your way into a more plant-based way of eating? Swap out half the ground pork for firm tofu. Or go all vegan and replace the pork with tofu. You can keep this dish light by serving it as-is. For a more substantial meal, serve it with brown rice.

1 tablespoon sesame oil

1 garlic clove

1-by- ½-inch piece fresh ginger, minced

½ cup shredded carrot

3 scallions, finely chopped

1 jalapeño pepper, finely chopped (optional)

1 pound ground pork

2 tablespoons reduced-sodium soy sauce (or gluten-free tamari, if desired)

1 tablespoon rice vinegar (unseasoned)

1 head Bibb lettuce

1 English cucumber, finely diced, for serving

1 red bell pepper, finely chopped, for serving

½ cup fresh mint, coarsely chopped, for serving

½ cup fresh basil, coarsely chopped, for serving

1. Heat the sesame oil in a large skillet over medium heat. Add the garlic, ginger, carrot, scallions, jalapeño (if using), pork, soy sauce, and vinegar. Cook for 5 minutes, or until the meat is cooked through. You may need to drain the skillet if your pork is particularly fatty.

2. Separate the lettuce leaves, wash, and keep the leaves whole.

3. To assemble the wraps, scoop the pork with the lettuce leaves. Garnish with the rest of the ingredients.

Ingredient tip: Nothing gives flavor like fresh herbs. Buy them in the supermarket or, better yet, grow them in your garden, in pots on your balcony, or even in a windowsill garden. What really elevates these wraps are the garnishes. For some extra flavor, try adding some fresh cilantro and freshly squeezed lime juice. Add a few peanuts for a bit of crunch and finish off with a sprinkle of sesame seeds.

PER SERVING: Calories: 432; Total fat: 32g; Total carbohydrates: 14g; Fiber: 4g; Protein: 24g; Sodium: 404mg

Pork Chops with Asparagus and Yams

GLUTEN-FREE

SERVES 4 / PREP TIME: 5 MINUTES / COOK TIME: 25 MINUTES

I love a meal that creates a minimum number of dirty dishes. This meal is amazingly easy to prepare, and you get a fully balanced meal with only one pan to wash up. How great is that? Pork pairs well with sweeter ingredients. In this recipe, I've paired it with naturally sweet yams (sweet potatoes). The asparagus rounds out this meal and provides an attractive (and healthy) green for your plate.

2 tablespoons plus 1 teaspoon extra-virgin olive oil, divided

3 cups yams, peeled and diced

4 cups asparagus, cut into 2-inch lengths

1 teaspoon chili powder

1 teaspoon cumin

1 teaspoon paprika

½ teaspoon ground coriander

½ teaspoon garlic powder

1 teaspoon salt

½ teaspoon ground black pepper

4 boneless pork chops, 1-inch thick

1. Preheat the oven to 425°F.
2. Spread 2 tablespoons of oil on a sheet pan. Add the veggies and toss to coat in the oil. Then move them to one half of the pan.
3. In a small bowl, combine the spices. Sprinkle half the spice mixture on a plate. Place the pork chops on the plate to cover the underside in the spices. Then place the pork chops on the sheet pan, spiced-side down. Coat the top of each pork chop in the remaining spice mixture. Drizzle the pork chops with the remaining 1 teaspoon of olive oil.
4. Bake until a thermometer inserted in the pork reads 145°F and the asparagus and yams are tender, about 20 to 25 minutes. Let the pork stand 5 minutes before serving. To serve, divide all the ingredients among 4 serving plates.

Ingredient tip: Choose thicker asparagus for this recipe, so it takes the same amount of time to cook as the pork and yams.

PER SERVING: Calories: 366; Total fat: 15g; Total carbohydrates: 36g; Fiber: 3g; Protein: 26g; Sodium: 849mg

Pork Tenderloin with White Wine Sauce

GLUTEN-FREE

SERVES 4 / PREP TIME: 10 MINUTES / COOK TIME: 30 MINUTES

This elegant dish will impress any dinner guests. You don't need to tell them just how easy it is to prepare. Tenderloin is the most tender cut of pork (hence the name), so you really don't need to do much to it. In fact, it does best with a gentle hand, such as in this recipe. Impress your guests by serving the tenderloin with wild rice and steamed asparagus.

2 teaspoons dried oregano

1 teaspoon dried rosemary

¼ teaspoon dried thyme

¼ teaspoon salt

¼ teaspoon ground black pepper

1 pound pork tenderloin

1 tablespoon extra-virgin olive oil

¾ cup white wine

1 tablespoon unsalted butter

1. Preheat the oven to 400°F.

2. In a small bowl, combine the oregano, rosemary, thyme, salt, and pepper.

3. Trim the tenderloin of any silverskin. (This can be tough when cooked. Use a small knife and slide the blade under the silverskin to remove it.) Pat the pork dry with paper towels.

4. Heat the oil in a large oven-safe skillet (cast iron works well) over medium heat. Add the pork tenderloin and cook, turning occasionally, until browned all over, for 3 minutes total. Scatter the seasoning blend over the pork.

5. Transfer the skillet to the oven. Roast the tenderloin for 15 minutes, or until an internal thermometer inserted into the thickest part registers between 145°F and 150°F.

6. Transfer the pork to a large plate and cover with foil. Let it rest for 10 minutes.

Continued

Pork Tenderloin with White Wine Sauce Continued

7. While the pork is resting, put the skillet back over medium heat. Be sure to use an oven mitt as the handle will be searing hot. Add the white wine and simmer over medium heat until reduced by half. Add the butter.

8. Cut the pork into ¾-inch medallions. Divide among the serving plates and drizzle with the white wine sauce.

Ingredient tip: Pork tenderloin is different than pork loin. Tenderloin will be long and narrow, almost cylindrical in shape.

PER SERVING: Calories: 208; Total fat: 9g; Total carbohydrates: 2g; Fiber: 0g; Protein: 24g; Sodium: 218mg

Sausage and Pepper Pasta

GLUTEN-FREE (OPTION)

SERVES 4 / PREP TIME: 5 MINUTES / COOK TIME 20 MINUTES

In my opinion, a good pasta is a simple pasta, a delicious pairing of a few ingredients that really sing together. To save time when making pasta, gather and prepare your ingredients while you're bringing your water to a boil. Any shape pasta noodle works for this recipe, but my preference is a short noodle, such as rotini or penne. This recipe also makes a great pasta salad, so feel free to double the recipe in order to create leftovers.

12 ounces whole wheat pasta (gluten-free pasta, if desired)

1 red onion

2 red bell peppers

2 yellow bell peppers

8 cups spinach, packed

4 Italian sausages

2 tablespoons extra-virgin olive oil

2 garlic cloves, minced

1½ tablespoons chili powder

½ cup balsamic vinegar

¼ teaspoon ground black pepper

1. Bring a large pot of water to a boil over high heat. Add the pasta and cook until al dente, about 8 minutes.
2. Slice the onion and cut the bell peppers into strips. Coarsely chop the spinach. Cut the sausage into bite-size pieces.
3. Heat the oil in a large skillet over medium heat. Add the onions and sausage. Sauté for 2 minutes. Add the garlic and sauté for 30 seconds. Add the bell peppers, chili powder, vinegar, and pepper and sauté until the sausage and peppers are cooked, about 5 minutes.
4. Drain the pasta and toss with the sausage mixture. To serve, divide among 4 serving plates.

Ingredient tip: If you like a little heat, choose a hot Italian-style sausage. If you don't like the heat, choose a mild Italian sausage.

PER SERVING: Calories: 636; Total fat: 29g; Total carbohydrates: 85g; Fiber: 15g; Protein: 25g; Sodium: 580mg

Jenefer's Chili Con Carne

GLUTEN-FREE, MAKES GREAT LEFTOVERS

SERVES 8 / PREP TIME: 10 MINUTES / COOK TIME: 90 MINUTES

No, that's not a typo; the spelling of my mom's name is "Jenefer." I grew up eating this chili. It's so good that I've never had a chili that's even come close to it. My mom learned this recipe in a cooking class that she attended while living in Colorado in the 1970s. To truly make this recipe like my Mum does, you need to use pinto beans. Other beans will work if you can't find pinto beans. Just don't call it Jenefer's Chili if you use kidney beans. My mom detests kidney beans.

1 yellow onion

1 garlic clove

2 green bell peppers

4 hot chile peppers, dried, fresh, or frozen

3 tablespoons extra-virgin olive oil

1½ pounds lean ground beef

2 (15½-ounce) cans pinto beans

1 (28-ounce) can diced tomatoes

3 cups water

3 bay leaves

3 tablespoons chili powder

¼ teaspoon salt

1. Finely dice the onion, mince the garlic, and dice the bell peppers. Finely dice the chile peppers.
2. Heat the oil in a large stock pot over medium heat. Add the beef, onion, garlic, bell peppers, and chile peppers. Sauté until the meat has browned, about 4 minutes.
3. Add the beans, tomatoes, water, bay leaves, chili powder, and salt to the pot. Cover and simmer for at least an hour, stirring occasionally. The longer you simmer the chili, the more the flavor will develop.
4. To serve, divide among 4 serving bowls.

Storage tip: This recipe tastes even better as leftovers. Refrigerate as much as you will eat in the next 3 or 4 days. Freeze the remainder. It will keep for 2 or 3 months.

PER SERVING: Calories: 320; Total fat: 14g; Total carbohydrates: 26g; Fiber: 8g; Protein: 24g; Sodium: 472mg

Beef and Broccoli Stir-Fry

GLUTEN-FREE (OPTION), MAKE AHEAD

SERVES 4 / PREP TIME: 10 MINUTES / COOK TIME: 10 MINUTES

This recipe mimics the classic Chinese takeout dish but without any added sugar (or MSG). Almost every bottled stir-fry sauce on supermarket shelves contains free sugars. I say "almost" every bottle because there are some (hard to find) brands that do not have any free sugar. In this recipe, you are freed from bottled sauces.

½ cup plus 4 tablespoons water, divided

5 tablespoons cornstarch, divided

⅓ cup reduced-sodium soy sauce (or gluten-free tamari, if desired)

2-by-2-inch piece of fresh ginger, minced

1 teaspoon sesame oil

1 pound flank steak or stir-fry beef

1 tablespoon vegetable oil

½ yellow onion, sliced

1 chile pepper

8 cups broccoli, cut into small florets

2 garlic cloves, minced

4 cups cooked brown rice

4 tablespoons sesame seeds, divided

1. In a small bowl, combine ½ cup water, 1 tablespoon of cornstarch, soy sauce, ginger, and sesame oil. Stir until it is smooth. Set aside.

2. Slice the steak into strips. In a medium bowl, combine 4 tablespoons of cornstarch and 4 tablespoons of water. Add the beef and toss to coat.

3. Heat the vegetable oil in a large sauté pan or skillet over medium heat. Add the onion and chile and cook for 2 minutes. Add the broccoli and garlic and sauté for 3 or 4 minutes. Add the beef and sauté for 2 minutes, stirring frequently. Add the soy sauce mixture and cook for 4 minutes, or until desired level of doneness is achieved and the sauce has thickened.

4. To serve, divide the warm brown rice and stir fry among 4 serving bowls and garnish with 1 tablespoon of sesame seeds per serving.

Ingredient tip: Make your prep even faster with pre cut ingredients. Look for stir-fry beef (beef already cut into strips) and broccoli already cut into florets. Remove the seeds from the chile pepper if you don't like a bit of heat.

PER SERVING: Calories: 589; Total fat: 19g; Total carbohydrates: 69g; Fiber: 10g; Protein: 37g; Sodium: 835mg

TIME-SAVING MEAL PREP HACKS

Use the following meal prep hacks to maximize the time you spend in the kitchen.

Chop, chop. Need half an onion for tonight's dinner? Dice the full onion and save half for the next recipe. Does your recipe tonight call for sliced carrots? Cut some extra carrots into sticks for tomorrow's snack. Plan recipes that use similar ingredients. For example, both the Beef Fajitas (page 107) and Clam Linguini (page 122) include red bell peppers. Plan to make these dishes two days in a row and cut up enough bell peppers on day one for both dishes.

Buy prechopped. Food companies are really upping their game. It seems like every time that I'm in the supermarket, I find new vegetables that are preprepared to save you time. For example, there is garlic already minced, mushrooms already sliced, cabbage already shredded, and broccoli cut into spears. The frozen food section is also improving. For example, there are Brussels sprouts already washed and sliced, and butternut squash already cut into cubes (that's a big job).

Cook extra. When you have extra time, make big batch meals and freeze them in portions, such as Split Pea Soup with Ham (page 96). For foods that take longer to prepare, cook extra portions, then freeze. For example, brown rice freezes well. Make Lemon-Garlic Roast Chicken (page 91) and use the leftovers for other lunches and dinners, such as Classic Cobb Salad (page 49) or Chicken Soup with Quinoa (page 86).

Beef Fajitas

GLUTEN-FREE

SERVES 4 / TOTAL TIME: 20 MINUTES

Fajitas bring fun to even the most boring Tuesday night. I think it's the bright colors of the bell peppers, the ability to top it with your own personalized combination of toppings, and the opportunity to eat with your hands. You can make this recipe even quicker if you have some leftover cooked steak from a previous dinner, such as Pan-Seared Steak with Carrot-Parsnip Mash (page 108). At my local supermarket, they sell stir-fry beef that is already cut into strips. It's perfect for this recipe. Keep an eye out for it at your supermarket.

2 tablespoons chili powder

2 tablespoons dried oregano

¼ teaspoon cayenne

1 teaspoon cumin

1 pound flank steak or stir-fry beef

1 tablespoon vegetable oil

1 red onion, sliced

2 green bell peppers, sliced

2 red bell peppers, sliced

8 small (6-inch) corn tortillas , for serving

1 avocado, sliced, for serving (optional)

1 jar salsa, for serving (optional)

Sour cream or plain yogurt, for serving (optional)

Hot sauce, for serving (optional)

24 sprigs cilantro, for garnish (optional)

1 lime, quartered, for garnish (optional)

1. In a medium bowl, combine the chili powder, oregano, cayenne, and cumin. Slice the steak into strips. Add the steak to the spice mixture and toss to coat it evenly in the spices.

2. Heat the oil in a skillet over medium heat. Add the onion and cook for 1 minute. Then add in the bell peppers. Cook for 1 minute, stirring.

3. Move the vegetables to one side of your skillet. Add the meat and spices to the empty half. Sauté, stirring, until the meat is cooked through, about 7 minutes.

4. Assemble your fajitas using the tortillas to your desired specifications.

Equipment tip: I find tongs to be the best utensil for stirring the bell peppers and steak and for removing cooked items from the skillet.

PER SERVING: Calories: 407; Total fat: 13g; Total carbohydrates: 43g; Fiber: 5g; Protein: 28g; Sodium: 158mg

Pan-Seared Steak with Carrot-Parsnip Mash

GLUTEN-FREE, MAKES GREAT LEFTOVERS

SERVES 4 / PREP TIME: 10 MINUTES / COOK TIME: 25 MINUTES

A steak cooked on an outdoor grill is a beautiful thing, but we don't all have access to an outdoor grill. Whether you do or not, it's still good to know how to pan-sear a steak. Here, I've paired the steak with a carrot and parsnip mash. Parsnips are inexpensive veggies that many people overlook. Parsnips and carrots are a match made in heaven, so I encourage you to try this recipe as your introduction to parsnips.

FOR THE STEAK

2 teaspoons extra-virgin olive oil

Salt

Freshly ground black pepper

4 sirloin steaks, at least ¾-inch thick

3 tablespoons unsalted butter

2 peeled garlic cloves, left whole

FOR THE CARROT-PARSNIP MASH

4 cups diced carrots

4 cups diced parsnips

2 tablespoons unsalted butter

½ teaspoon salt

½ teaspoon ground black pepper

TO MAKE THE STEAK

1. Heat the oil in a large skillet over medium heat (do not use a nonstick pan).

2. Add salt and pepper to one side of the steaks.

3. Add the steaks, seasoned-side down. Salt and pepper the other side of the steaks. Do not move the steaks in the skillet for 2 minutes. Using tongs, flip the steaks and add the butter and garlic to the skillet. With a spoon, keep basting the melted butter over the steaks. Baste continually (tilt the pan a little if you have to, to get the butter onto the spoon). You've likely seen this technique if you've ever watched a TV cooking show.

4. Remove from the heat at about the 4- or 5-minute mark of total cooking time for a medium-rare steak. Cook a minute or two longer for medium to well-done. A thicker steak may take longer.

5. Turn off the heat and baste one more time. Remove to a plate and cover with another plate, flipped upside down, or with foil. Leave the steaks covered for 10 minutes and allow to rest before cutting.

TO MAKE THE CARROT-PARSNIP MASH

1. Fill a large saucepan with water. Cover and bring to a boil over high heat.
2. Add the carrots and parsnips to the pot of water.
3. Cook 15 minutes, or until the veggies are soft.
4. Drain in a colander and return to the pot. Add the butter, salt, and pepper. Mash.

Equipment tip: An immersion blender is the best tool to mash the carrots and parsnips, but a potato masher will work.

PER SERVING: Calories: 493; Total fat: 27g; Total carbohydrates: 39g; Fiber: 9g; Protein: 25g; Sodium: 494mg

Muffin Tin Mini Meat Loaves

GLUTEN-FREE (OPTION), MAKES GREAT LEFTOVERS

SERVES 9 / PREP TIME: 15 MINUTES / COOK TIME: 20 MINUTES

I love a classic meat loaf. It's good, old-fashioned comfort food. But traditional loaves take 1 or 2 hours to cook—far too long for a weeknight meal. Here, I use a trusty muffin tin to transform meat loaf into a quick weeknight dinner option. Pair the meat loaf with some steamed carrots and mashed yams to round out this comfort food favorite. If you like meat loaf, you likely know that it always tastes better the next day, so this recipe makes plenty of leftovers.

1½ cups rolled oats (gluten-free, if desired)

½ cup milk

1 cup tomato juice

2 eggs

1 yellow onion, finely diced

2 pounds lean ground beef

1 tablespoon dried parsley

½ teaspoon dried thyme

¼ teaspoon salt

2 teaspoons ground black pepper

Cooking oil spray

1. Preheat the oven to 350°F.
2. In a medium bowl, soak the oats in the milk and tomato juice.
3. In a large bowl, beat the eggs. Add the oat mixture, onion, beef, parsley, thyme, salt, and pepper. Mix thoroughly with your hands to combine the ingredients.
4. Generously spray a muffin tin with cooking oil spray, both the bottom and sides of the depressions. Fill to the top with the meat mix.
5. Bake for 20 minutes.
6. Allow to cool for 5 minutes before removing from the muffin tin.
7. For the second batch of 6 muffins, add a splash of water to the empty muffin cups.

Storage tip: Store your mini meat loaves in the refrigerator for 3 or 4 days or in the freezer for 2 or 3 months.

PER SERVING: Calories: 347; Total fat: 23g; Total carbohydrates: 12g; Fiber: 2g; Protein: 22g; Sodium: 233mg

Hamburgers with Hidden Veggies

GLUTEN-FREE (OPTION)

SERVES 4 / PREP TIME: 15 MINUTES / COOK TIME: 10 MINUTES

Okay, calling the spinach in these burgers "hidden" may be a bit of a stretch. You will be able to see the spinach, but you won't taste it or experience its texture because it's totally overwhelmed by the burger. If you struggle to eat leafy greens, then this recipe makes it easy. Serve these burgers on a whole wheat bun with your favorite toppings, such as lettuce, tomato, and onion.

2 tablespoons butter, divided

4 cups chopped spinach

2 egg yolks

1 pound lean ground beef

½ cup finely diced onion

⅛ teaspoon salt

¼ teaspoon ground black pepper

4 whole wheat hamburger buns (gluten-free, if desired)

2 tomatoes, sliced, for garnish

Lettuce, for garnish (optional)

Red onion, sliced, for garnish (optional)

Mustard, for garnish (optional)

1. In a skillet, melt 1 tablespoon of the butter over medium heat. Add the spinach, in batches if necessary, and cook until wilted, about 1 minute.

2. Put the yolks in a large bowl. Whisk with a fork. Add the beef, onion, salt, pepper, and the cooked spinach. Mix thoroughly with your hands and form four burger patties.

3. Stovetop method: If sautéing the burgers, make flat patties. In a skillet over medium heat, melt 1 tablespoon of the butter. Sauté the burgers for 10 minutes, flipping once about halfway through.

4. Grill method: Preheat the grill on medium heat. Grill the burgers, 3 minutes per side, closing the lid while grilling.

5. Serve on whole wheat buns with your desired garnishes.

Ingredient tip: Read the labels carefully on your burger condiments. Barbeque sauce and ketchup both contain free sugar. Mustard and mayonnaise are good choices.

PER SERVING: Calories: 565; Total fat: 35g; Total carbohydrates: 37g; Fiber: 9g; Protein: 30g; Sodium: 566mg

Peruvian Beef Sheet Pan Meal

GLUTEN-FREE (OPTION)

SERVES 4 / PREP TIME: 10 MINUTES / COOK TIME: 20 MINUTES

Peruvian food—particularly the food in Lima, Peru's largest city—is a fascinating combination of indigenous Peruvian, European (especially Spanish), African, Chinese, and Japanese cuisines. All these food traditions are combined to create a unique cuisine that is beyond chef-forced fusion fare. In this recipe, I combine the staples of indigenous Peru (tomatoes, potatoes, and chiles), soy sauce and ginger, as well as balsamic vinegar to bring a little bit of Lima to your dinner table.

2 tablespoons reduced-sodium soy sauce (or gluten-free tamari, if desired)

3 tablespoons balsamic vinegar

2 tablespoons finely minced ginger

1 chile pepper (e.g., jalapeño), diced (Omit seeds if you prefer a milder dish. Include seeds for more heat.)

½ teaspoon salt

½ teaspoon ground black pepper

1 pound sirloin tip steak

1 red onion

3 cups new potatoes, cut into ½-inch pieces

½ head garlic

2 tablespoons extra-virgin olive oil, divided

3 cups cherry tomatoes, halved

1. Preheat the oven to 375°F.
2. In a medium bowl, combine the soy sauce, balsamic vinegar, ginger, chile pepper, salt, and pepper. Add the steak to marinate while you prepare the rest of the dish.
3. Cut the red onion into 8 wedges. Cut the potatoes into ½-inch pieces. Remove the outer skin (the loose stuff) from the garlic and break the head into individual cloves. Do not peel or crush the cloves (leave them whole).
4. Pour 1 tablespoon of oil on a metal sheet pan. Add the potatoes, garlic, and onion. Toss them to coat in the oil, then move them to one corner of the pan.
5. Add the tomatoes to the pan. Drizzle 1 tablespoon of oil over them and toss gently to coat, then move them to one section of the pan. The veggies should be taking up ¾ of the space on the pan.
6. Add the steak to the free edge of the pan, pouring the marinade over the steak.
7. Roast for 20 minutes. Remove the steak and transfer it to a plate. Cover the steak with another plate, flipped upside down (like a sandwich), or cover with foil to allow it to rest. Return the sheet pan to the oven and cook for 5 more minutes.

8. To serve, cut the steak in two. Divide the steak and veggies between two plates.

Cooking tip: These directions created a medium steak. If you prefer your steak medium-rare, allow the vegetable mixture to cook for 5 minutes before adding the steak to the sheet pan, then roast for 15 minutes.

PER SERVING: Calories: 302; Total fat: 13g; Total carbohydrates: 19g; Fiber: 3g; Protein: 24g; Sodium: 934mg

7

FISH & SEAFOOD

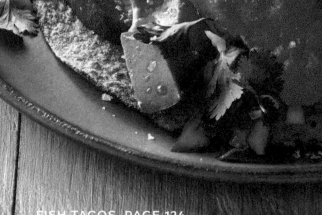

FISH TACOS, PAGE 124

Seafood Cioppino

GLUTEN-FREE, MAKES GREAT LEFTOVERS

SERVES 6 / TOTAL TIME: 1 HOUR

This is an Italian version of a tomato-based seafood chowder. You can mix and match the seafood in this chowder, such as adding scallops and using cod instead of the tilapia. I recommend keeping the chile pepper, even if you don't like spicy food. You can include the flesh of the pepper but omit the seeds, as the seeds provide most of the heat in a chile pepper. This dish isn't intended to blow your head off—the heat is a subtle touch.

¼ cup extra-virgin olive oil

2 green bell peppers, diced

1 yellow onion, diced

1 chile pepper, finely diced

4 garlic cloves

1 (28-ounce) can diced tomatoes

1 (15-ounce) can tomato sauce

1 cup water

1 cup white wine

1 (10-ounce) can clams, with their liquid

1 cup diced fresh flat-leaf Italian parsley

1 tablespoon dried basil

1 tablespoon dried oregano

1 teaspoon paprika

¼ teaspoon cayenne

¼ teaspoon salt

½ teaspoon ground black pepper

2 tilapia fillets

25 medium to large shrimp , deveined

25 mussels

1. Heat the oil in a large saucepan over medium heat. Add the green peppers, onion, and chile pepper. Sauté, stirring frequently, until the onion is translucent, about 4 minutes. Add the garlic. Sauté, stirring constantly, for 1 minute.

2. Add the tomatoes, tomato sauce, water, wine, juice from the clams, parsley, basil, oregano, paprika, cayenne, salt, and pepper.

3. Cover. Increase the heat to high and bring to a boil.

4. Lower the heat to medium and cook, covered, for 15 minutes, stirring occasionally.

5. Prepare the seafood. Cut the tilapia into 1-inch pieces. Peel the shrimp and remove their tails. Rinse, clean, and debeard the mussels. Add the tilapia, shrimp, mussels, and clams to the chowder. Cook for 10 minutes.

6. To serve, divide among 6 serving bowls.

Storage tip: Store leftovers in the refrigerator. Eat them within 3 or 4 days.

PER SERVING: Calories: 424; Total fat: 14g; Total carbohydrates: 26g; Fiber: 5g; Protein: 44g; Sodium: 1,444mg

HOW TO SAFELY THAW FROZEN FISH

Following these methods minimizes any risk of foodborne illness (commonly called food poisoning) when defrosting frozen fish and other seafood. Each of these methods promotes even thawing, which minimizes bacteria growth, thus minimizing any risk.

But before I cover the different methods to defrost your fish, we need to talk about vacuum packages. To create the best quality, fish are often sealed in vacuum packages before being frozen. Bacteria can grow inside the sealed packages while defrosting. Therefore, always remove fish from vacuum packaging before defrosting, no matter which defrost method you choose.

Refrigerator method: This is the easiest method. It is also the preferred method for having the best quality fish. Simply put the frozen fish in the refrigerator the night before you plan to eat it. Your fish will slowly defrost in time for dinner. I recommend placing your fish in a bowl or on a plate with a rim to catch any juices that may be released while it defrosts.

If you forgot to take the seafood out of the freezer last night, you can use either of these two methods:

Cool water method: Put your seafood in a sealed plastic bag and immerse it in cold water.

Microwave method: Only use this method if you will be cooking the seafood immediately after defrosting it. Microwave your seafood on the defrost setting. Stop defrosting when the fish is still icy but pliable.

Lemon-Garlic Shrimp Kebabs

GLUTEN-FREE

SERVES 4 / PREP TIME: 15 MINUTES / COOK TIME: 10 MINUTES

Here in Canada, we call medium and large shrimp "prawns." Whether you call them shrimp or prawns, they're delicious in this simple kebab recipe. It's a quick and delicious recipe for rushed weeknights, and it makes a pretty dinner party meal—just double or triple the recipe. I mean, who doesn't love dipping seafood in garlic butter? Unlike most kebab recipes, I find that this one works best in the oven, so I didn't include cooking instructions for a grill.

8 skewers, metal or wooden

Cooking oil spray

3 lemons, divided

3 orange bell peppers

32 medium to large shrimp

¼ cup unsalted butter

4 garlic cloves, minced

¼ cup chopped fresh parsley leaves

⅛ teaspoon salt

⅛ teaspoon ground black pepper

1. Preheat the oven to 450°F.
2. If using wooden skewers, put them in a large shallow dish and soak them in water while you prepare the remaining ingredients.
3. Coat a sheet pan with the cooking oil spray.
4. Cut 2 lemons into half-moon slices as wide as your shrimp. Cut the bell peppers into 1-inch pieces.
5. Peel and devein the shrimp.
6. Assemble the shrimp, bell peppers, and lemons on the skewers.
7. Place the skewers onto the prepared baking sheet. Put in the oven and roast until cooked through, about 7 minutes.
8. Juice the remaining lemon and set aside.
9. Melt the butter in a medium skillet over medium-high heat. Stir in the lemon juice, garlic, fresh parsley, salt, and pepper. Sauté, stirring, for 2 minutes or until the sauce is fragrant. Transfer the sauce into a serving bowl.

10. Serve the skewers immediately with the garlic butter dipping sauce.

Storage tip: To store leftovers, remove the shrimp, lemons, and bell peppers from the skewers. Discard the lemon slices. Store shrimp and bell peppers in the refrigerator for 3 or 4 days. This recipe doesn't freeze well.

PER SERVING: Calories: 227; Total fat: 12g; Total carbohydrates: 18g; Fiber: 6g; Protein: 19g; Sodium: 582mg

Thai Coconut Fish Curry

GLUTEN-FREE, MAKE AHEAD, MAKES GREAT LEFTOVERS

SERVES 4 / PREP TIME: 10 MINUTES / COOK TIME: 15 MINUTES

Thai curry paste is just about the only jarred sauce in the Asian food section of your supermarket that doesn't contain free sugars. When buying curry paste, I always have to stop and think it through. You see, the colors of the curry paste indicate the level of heat, but in the opposite direction my intuition would tell me. Red curry is the mildest curry. Yellow curry is in the middle. Green curry is the hottest. Choose the paste that best matches your heat preference. Serve this curry on top of brown rice.

4 tilapia fillets

1 tablespoon vegetable oil

½ yellow onion, diced

1 green bell pepper, medium diced

3 cups bok choy, roughly chopped

1½ cups sliced mushrooms

1 (13½-ounce) can full-fat coconut milk

2½ tablespoons Thai curry paste (red, yellow, or green)

1½ cups bean sprouts

4 cups cooked brown rice

½ cup fresh cilantro, chopped, for garnish

1. Cut the tilapia into 1-inch pieces.

2. Heat the oil in a large skillet over low-medium heat. Add the onions and sauté until the onions are translucent, about 4 minutes. Increase the heat to medium. Add the bell peppers, bok choy, mushrooms, coconut milk, curry paste, and tilapia. Sauté, stirring frequently, until the fish and veggies are cooked, about 10 minutes. Add the bean sprouts in the final 2 minutes of cooking.

3. To serve, put 1 cup of rice into each bowl. Divide the curry among the 4 bowls, putting it on top of the rice. Garnish with the cilantro.

Ingredient tip: A lot of the flavor compounds in the curry paste require fat to really come alive. For this reason, I recommend using regular (not low-fat) coconut milk.

PER SERVING: Calories: 577; Total fat: 24g; Total carbohydrates: 58g; Fiber: 7g; Protein: 33g; Sodium: 753mg

Simply Delicious Sautéed Shrimp

GLUTEN-FREE

SERVES 4 / PREP TIME: 10 MINUTES / COOK TIME: 5 MINUTES

Spot prawns are a shrimp local to the Pacific Northwest and are absolutely delicious. They have a very short season when they can be legally caught, usually starting in May. This is my go-to recipe during the short spot prawn season. It's such an elegant and delicate recipe for shrimp. It doesn't store well, so eat everything the day you make it. Pair it with a simple tossed salad and serve on top of rice, pouring the sauce over top of the rice, or serve in bowls and sop up the sauce with pieces of crusty artisan whole grain bread.

---

4 pounds medium to large shrimp

1 tablespoon unsalted butter

1 tablespoon extra-virgin olive oil

2 garlic cloves, minced

1 chile pepper, finely diced and most of the seeds removed

½ cup white wine

¼ cup fresh lemon juice (from 1 lemon)

⅛ teaspoon salt

⅛ teaspoon ground black pepper

1. Peel and devein the shrimp.
2. Melt the butter and oil together in a large skillet over medium heat. Add the shrimp, garlic, and chile pepper. Sauté, stirring, for 2 minutes. Add the wine, lemon juice, salt, and pepper. Sauté, stirring for 2 more minutes, or until the shrimp are pink and cooked.
3. Serve immediately by dividing the shrimp among 4 serving plates.

Ingredient tip: Most of the heat in a chile pepper is contained in the seeds. Removing most of the seeds allows the chile to provide its almost fruity sweetness to the dish with only a hint of heat.

PER SERVING: Calories: 365; Total fat: 6g; Total carbohydrates: 3g; Fiber: 0g; Protein: 68g; Sodium: 2,079mg

Clam Linguini

GLUTEN-FREE (OPTION)

SERVES 4 / TOTAL TIME: 30 MINUTES

Pasta is such a crowd-pleasing, quick weeknight meal. I think everyone should have a lot of pasta recipes in their repertoire. I've created a tasty pasta with the classic pairing of clams with sausage. Linguini noodles are called for in this recipe, but you can use any shaped pasta that you wish. Take care not to overcook the noodles. Cooking the noodles only until al dente lowers the pasta's glycemic index, meaning it will minimize any blood sugar spike.

12 ounces whole wheat linguini noodles (gluten-free, if desired)

1 teaspoon extra-virgin olive oil

1 chorizo sausage

1 shallot, diced

2 red bell peppers, sliced

2 garlic cloves, minced

⅛ teaspoon salt

¼ teaspoon ground black pepper

⅓ cup white wine

1 (6½-ounce) can clams, drained

6 cups spinach, coarsely chopped

1. Bring a large pot of water to a boil. Add the pasta. Cook until the pasta is al dente, about 6 minutes.
2. Cut the sausage into bite-size pieces.
3. Heat the oil in a large skillet over medium heat. Sauté the sausage for 1 minute. Add the shallot, bell peppers, garlic, salt, and pepper. Sauté for 2 minutes.
4. Add the wine and clams. Bring the sauce back up to a simmer. Add the spinach, in batches if necessary. Cook until the spinach has just wilted, about 2 minutes.
5. Drain the pasta and toss with the sauce. To serve, divide the pasta among 4 serving plates.

Ingredient tip: Shallots are a member of the onion family. They are smaller than your standard cooking onion and pink in color. They have a delicate flavor. Use red onion if you can't find shallots at your supermarket.

PER SERVING: Calories: 425; Total fat: 8g; Total carbohydrates: 71g; Fiber: 11g; Protein: 22g; Sodium: 236mg

Steamed Salmon with Asparagus and Leeks

GLUTEN-FREE

SERVES 4 / TOTAL TIME: 20 MINUTES

This dish is elegant in its simplicity. It's a perfect spring dish when asparagus comes into season. This recipe also works well for trout and delicate white fish, such as sole and tilapia. Choose thicker asparagus spears so they don't overcook before the fish is ready. You can double or triple the recipe (for leftovers or dinner parties) if you use bamboo steamer baskets. Simply stack the baskets one on top of the other, rotating them during the cooking time to achieve even steaming.

6 cups water

4 cups asparagus

1 leek

1 lemon

4 salmon fillets

⅛ teaspoon salt

⅛ teaspoon ground black pepper

1. In a large saucepan, bring the water to a boil.
2. Snap the tough ends off of the asparagus and lay them down to cover the bottom of a steamer basket. Slice the leek and lay it on top of the asparagus. Slice the lemon and lay it on top of the leeks.
3. Lay the salmon fillets on top of the bed of lemon slices. Season with salt and pepper.
4. Cover and steam, 10 minutes per inch of thickness of your fish.

Equipment tip: Use a metal steamer basket or two bamboo baskets (like those found in dim sum restaurants) stacked on top of each other. You can find inexpensive bamboo baskets online.

PER SERVING: Calories: 280; Total fat: 14g; Total carbohydrates: 12g; Fiber: 4g; Protein: 29g; Sodium: 151mg

Fish Tacos

GLUTEN-FREE (OPTION)

SERVES 4 / PREP TIME: 5 MINUTES / COOK TIME: 10 MINUTES

This is a very simple fish taco recipe. It's perfect for my absolute favorite fish: halibut. If you can't find halibut in your local supermarket or your price range (halibut is expensive), you can substitute other white fish such as cod. Even salmon works in this recipe. Be sure to use a large skillet and don't be tempted to use less oil for frying. Be patient and wait until your oil is truly hot before adding the fish to your skillet. Not waiting will result in soggy fish, and no one wants a soggy fish taco.

½ cup all-purpose flour (gluten-free, if desired)

½ teaspoon plus a pinch salt, divided

½ teaspoon plus ⅛ teaspoon ground black pepper, divided

2 pounds firm white fish, such as halibut or cod, cut into 2-inch chunks

⅓ cup vegetable oil

3 cups cabbage, shredded

2 tablespoons lime juice, plus additional for garnish

1 teaspoon extra-virgin olive oil

1 avocado

8 corn hard taco shells (or 6-inch tortillas)

¼ cup chopped cilantro, for garnish

Hot sauce, for garnish (optional)

1. Combine the flour, ½ teaspoon salt, and ½ teaspoon pepper on a plate with a rim. Pat the fish dry with a paper towel. Dredge both sides of the fish fillets in the flour mixture.

2. Heat the oil in large skillet over medium-high heat. Add the fish. Sauté, until the fish is browned on all sides, about 10 minutes.

3. Put the shredded cabbage in a small bowl. Add the lime juice, olive oil, a pinch of salt, and ⅛ teaspoon pepper. Toss to evenly coat the cabbage in the dressing.

4. Slice the avocado.

5. Assemble your tacos. Top each with the fish, cabbage, and avocado. Garnish with cilantro, hot sauce (if using), and an additional squeeze of fresh lime juice.

Ingredient tip: Using preshredded cabbage, often sold as coleslaw mix, is a fantastic time saver.

PER SERVING: Calories: 705; Total fat: 36g; Total carbohydrates: 27g; Fiber: 5g; Protein: 64g; Sodium: 499mg

FRESH, FROZEN, CANNED

When it comes to choosing the best seafood, fresh isn't always best. Well—let me back up a bit. Fresh is the best. But often, the freshest fish isn't where you think it'd be.

Often, the freshest fish is hiding in the frozen or canned food sections. I'm lucky to have fish stores in my neighborhood where I can buy fish that came off the boat that same day, but sometimes I don't have the time (or budget) to do this extra shopping. Here are tips to find the best quality fish in any supermarket—whether you live on an island in the Pacific Ocean or in the middle of the Nebraska prairie.

Frozen. Modern fishing boats are amazing. Many are equipped so that the fish is flash frozen on board, immediately after being caught. This means that the fish is incredibly fresh and the best possible quality, even though it's frozen.

Canned. Canning stations are built on the coast in order for the fish to be incredibly fresh when it's canned. Therefore, canned seafood can be a good quality and affordable choice. For example, did you know that the vast majority of canned salmon is wild salmon?

Salmon Cakes

GLUTEN-FREE (OPTION)

SERVES 4 / PREP TIME: 5 MINUTES / COOK TIME: 10 MINUTES

This is a favorite quick, easy recipe made using staple ingredients that you likely already have in your home. It's a good dinner on hot summer nights when you don't want to be sweating in the kitchen for too long. Serve a tossed salad and artisan whole grain bread alongside your salmon cakes to round out the meal. If you don't like removing the skin and crushing the bones in canned salmon, you can now buy canned salmon without any skin or bones.

½ cup whole grain cracker crumbs (gluten-free, if desired)

2 large eggs

1 (14.75-ounce) can salmon, skin removed and bones crushed

¼ teaspoon paprika

1½ tablespoons unsalted butter

1. Put 4 crackers in a sealable plastic bag. Crush into crumbs with your hands or a rolling pin.
2. In a medium-size bowl, beat the eggs. Add the cracker crumbs, canned salmon, and paprika. Mix well.
3. Heat a large sauté pan or skillet over medium-high heat. Melt a generous pat of butter in the pan.
4. With your hands, form the salmon mixture into cakes. Fry in the butter, flipping once, until both sizes are golden brown, about 8 minutes.
5. Serve immediately by dividing among 4 serving plates next to your sides.

Storage tip: This recipe makes a seemingly awkward 5 cakes—one cake per person and one leftover. However, the cakes are delicious served atop a salad for lunch. Store leftover salmon cakes in the refrigerator for 3 or 4 days.

PER SERVING: Calories: 220; Total fat: 10g; Total carbohydrates: 6g; Fiber: 0g; Protein: 28g; Sodium: 502mg

Halibut with Tropical Fruit Salsa

GLUTEN-FREE

SERVES 4 / COOK TIME: 10 MINUTES

Calling this recipe a salsa isn't really doing it justice. This is a refreshing salad to serve alongside your fish. As such, it's a perfect summertime meal. Add some leftover brown rice or artisan whole grain bread and you've got a balanced meal. Any firm white fish works in this recipe, such as swordfish. It also is delicious with a tuna steak. Feel free to adjust any of the ingredients in the salsa. Love mango? Double the mango and omit the pineapple. Like spicy food? Include a chile pepper, such as jalapeño.

1 tablespoon extra-virgin olive oil

4 halibut fillets

⅛ teaspoon plus a pinch salt, divided

⅛ teaspoon plus a pinch ground black pepper, divided

1 cup diced cucumber (½ of an English cucumber)

1 cup diced red bell pepper

½ cup diced red onion

1 fresh chile pepper, finely diced (optional)

½ avocado, diced

½ cup mango, diced

½ cup pineapple, diced

¼ cup fresh cilantro, chopped

¼ cup fresh mint, chopped

2 tablespoons lime juice

1. Heat the oil in a large skillet over medium heat. Put the fish in the pan, skin-side down. Season with a pinch of salt and black pepper. Sauté until the fish flakes, 10 minutes per inch of fish, flipping the fillets three-quarters of the way through the cooking time.
2. Dice and chop all of the vegetables, fruit, and herbs.
3. In a medium bowl, combine the vegetables, fruit, fresh herbs, lime juice, ⅛ teaspoon salt, and ⅛ teaspoon pepper.
4. Serve the fish alongside your refreshing salsa.

Storage tip: You can easily double this recipe to make leftovers. Note that the salsa doesn't freeze well. Store the salsa in your refrigerator separate from the fish. Eat within 3 or 4 days (the salsa is best when eaten within 2 days).

PER SERVING: Calories: 262; Total fat: 8g; Total carbohydrates: 15g; Fiber: 4g; Protein: 36g; Sodium: 77mg

Sole Roll-Ups

MAKE AHEAD

SERVES 4 / PREP TIME: 20 MINUTES / COOK TIME: 20 MINUTES

Sole is so thin that it can easily become dry. In this recipe, it is stuffed with spinach and bread crumbs and poached in white wine and lemon juice, making for moist fish. Sole is a very mild fish (it doesn't have much fishy flavor), so it's a great starting point if you're new to eating seafood. Most store-bought bread crumbs contain free sugar. To make your own bread crumbs, leave 4 slices of whole wheat bread out overnight to harden. Cut off the crusts. Put them in a large resealable plastic bag and crumble with your hands or a rolling pin.

FOR THE BREAD CRUMBS

1 cup dry bread crumbs

¾ cup shredded Parmesan cheese

1 cup fresh Italian parsley, chopped

Zest from 1 lemon

3 teaspoons dried oregano

8 tablespoons extra-virgin olive oil

FOR THE SOLE

2 tablespoons butter

Juice from 1 lemon

1 cup white wine

12 boneless, skinless sole fillets

36 leaves spinach

1. Preheat the oven to 350°F.
2. In a small bowl, mix together the bread crumbs, Parmesan cheese, parsley, lemon zest, oregano, and olive oil.
3. Coat the bottom of a 9-by-13-inch glass lasagna pan with the butter. Add the lemon juice and white wine to the pan.
4. Lay the fish on a flat work surface. Line each fillet with 3 leaves of spinach. Top with a thin line of the bread crumb mixture. Roll up each fillet. Insert a toothpick to hold it securely. Place each fish roll-up in the baking dish.
5. Bake for about 20 minutes, or until the fish is cooked through.

Serving tip: Don't forget to remove the toothpick before serving.

PER SERVING: Calories: 683; Total fat: 49g; Total carbohydrates: 23g; Fiber: 2g; Protein: 30g; Sodium: 646mg

Asian-Style Fish in a Packet

GLUTEN-FREE (OPTION), MAKE AHEAD

SERVES 4 / PREP TIME: 10 MINUTES / COOK TIME: 10 MINUTES

Cooking fish in a tightly closed packet with veggies does two things. First, it makes dinner cleanup a breeze. Second, the closed packet keeps all the moisture inside, resulting in very moist fish. This technique is endlessly adaptable. Mix and match your favorite fish, veggies, and seasonings. You can keep an Asian flavor profile with other Asian greens. Or go Mediterranean with garlic, oregano, orange slices, spinach, and fennel. Another option is to try it Mexican style with onions, bell peppers, cumin, and chiles.

4 teaspoons extra-virgin olive oil, divided

4 cups sliced mushrooms, divided

32 leaves baby bok choy

4 tilapia fillets

Black pepper

1 garlic clove, minced

2-by-1-inch piece of ginger, finely minced

4 teaspoons reduced-sodium soy sauce, divided (or gluten-free tamari, if desired)

4 cups cooked brown rice

1. Preheat the oven to 450°F.
2. On a flat work surface, put a piece of foil, shiny side facing up. Spread 1 teaspoon of oil around the middle of the foil. Arrange the mushrooms on the foil and put 8 leaves of baby bok choy on top. Place 1 fillet of tilapia on top of the baby bok choy. Sprinkle the fish with black pepper, ¼ the garlic, and ¼ the ginger. Sprinkle with 1 teaspoon of the soy sauce.
3. Fold up the foil to make a packet. Place on a sheet pan, fold-side up.
4. Repeat to create the remaining 3 packets.
5. Bake in the oven for 10 minutes per inch of thickness of fish. Be careful when opening, as it will release steam. Serve one packet per person along with 1 cup of the brown rice.

Ingredient tip: If you only use ginger on occasion, store it in the freezer. This will keep it fresh. And, if you allow it to only partially defrost before preparing, it's the perfect texture for peeling and mincing.

PER SERVING: Calories: 408; Total fat: 9g; Total carbohydrates: 51g; Fiber: 5g; Protein: 33g; Sodium: 279mg

Olive Oil–Poached Salmon with Orange and Fennel

GLUTEN-FREE

SERVES 4 / PREP TIME: 10 MINUTES / COOK TIME: 20 MINUTES

This is my favorite recipe in the whole cookbook. Shhh, don't tell the other recipes. Pairing fennel and oranges is common in southern Italian and Sicilian cuisines. Fennel can be expensive out of season. When it is in season or when I see it on sale in my local supermarket, I snap it up for this recipe. Serve this dish with some artisanal whole wheat bread for a special date-night meal with your loved one.

4 fennel bulbs

1 leek, sliced

Zest from 2 oranges

2 cups olive oil

2 cups vegetable oil

1 chile pepper, whole

2 bay leaves

4 salmon fillets

¼ teaspoon salt

¼ teaspoon ground black pepper

1. Quarter, core, and thinly slice the fennel. Slice the white part and tender light-green part of the leek. Zest the oranges.

2. In a medium saucepan, combine the fennel, leek, orange zest, oils, chile pepper, and bay leaves. Cover and bring to a boil over high heat. Lower the heat to medium and simmer, stirring occasionally, for 10 minutes.

3. Carefully lay the salmon fillets on top of the fennel mixture, spooning the oil over top. Cover and cook for 7 minutes.

4. Carefully remove the salmon fillets. Set aside.

5. WARNING: Be very careful when straining the fennel mixture. The oil is scalding hot. Allow the oil to cool before you handle it. Using a colander over a heatproof bowl (not plastic), strain the fennel mixture, squeezing to drain the oil.

6. Discard the bay leaf and chile pepper. Spoon the fennel mixture onto 4 plates. Top with the salmon and season with salt and pepper.

Ingredient tip: This recipe also works well with other types of fish, such as halibut or cod.

PER SERVING: Calories: 352; Total fat: 18g; Total carbohydrates: 21g; Fiber: 8g; Protein: 28g; Sodium: 342mg

Salmon, Zucchini, and Yam Sheet Pan Meal

GLUTEN-FREE

SERVES 4 / PREP TIME: 15 MINUTES / COOK TIME: 25 MINUTES

This recipe is endlessly adaptable. Mix and match your root veggies, such as potatoes, carrots, and parsnips. Any fish with its skin on works well, such as halibut or sole. Roast the fish for 10 minutes per inch of thickness of the fish. If your fish is much thinner or thicker than an inch, roast the vegetables for a shorter or longer amount of time before adding the fish, so that everything is ready at the same time. Dice the vegetables into small cubes, as larger-size veggies won't cook in time to be eaten with your fish.

1 head garlic

4 cups yams, peeled and diced in ¾-inch cubes

5 cups zucchini, diced in ¾-inch cubes

2 tablespoons plus 1 teaspoon extra-virgin olive oil, divided

⅛ teaspoon salt

¼ teaspoon ground black pepper

2 lemons, each cut into 4 slices

4 salmon fillets

1. Preheat the oven to 425°F.
2. Remove the outermost skin (the loose stuff) from the garlic and break it into individual cloves. Leave the cloves whole.
3. Put the garlic, yams, and zucchini on a sheet pan. Drizzle the olive oil over the top and toss to coat the vegetables. Season with the salt and pepper.
4. Spread the vegetables in one layer over the sheet pan. Roast for 15 minutes.
5. Remove the vegetables from the oven and stir. Then place the lemon slices over top of the vegetables, making a bed for the salmon. Place the salmon, skin-side down, on top of the lemon slices.
6. Brush the salmon with the remaining 1 teaspoon of oil.
7. Roast for 10 minutes, or until the fish flakes.

Storage tip: Fill your sheet pan with veggies. They make great leftovers. I particularly like them as a cold, roasted vegetable salad. Discard the lemon slices and store in the refrigerator for 3 or 4 days.

PER SERVING: Calories: 515; Total fat: 23g; Total carbohydrates: 54g; Fiber: 11g; Protein: 30g; Sodium: 236mg

Salmon with Lentils

GLUTEN-FREE

SERVES 4 / PREP TIME: 5 MINUTES / COOK TIME: 10 MINUTES

This dish pairs salmon with the earthy flavors of grainy mustard and lentils. The lemon zest provides the bright flavor needed to create balance. I love this dish served cold the next day. If you want to make leftovers, double the recipe and use a larger pan. A 9-by-13-inch pan works well, as does a baking sheet. In this recipe, the lentils take the place of rice, providing fiber and low-glycemic index steady energy.

2 (15½-ounce) can lentils

1 leek, white part only

1 tablespoon plus 4 teaspoons extra-virgin olive oil, divided

2 tablespoons lemon zest (from 2 lemons)

¼ teaspoon salt

¼ teaspoon ground black pepper

4 salmon fillets

4 tablespoons grainy mustard

1. Preheat the oven to 425°F.
2. Drain and rinse the lentils.
3. Slice the white part of the leek.
4. Pour 1 tablespoon of the oil in an 8-by-8-inch metal baking dish. Add the lentils, leek, lemon zest, salt, and pepper. Stir to combine. Spread the lentils in an even layer.
5. Place the salmon on the lentils, skin-side down.
6. In a small bowl, combine the mustard with 4 teaspoons of olive oil. Top salmon with the mustard mixture.
7. Roast for 10 minutes per inch of thickness of the fish.

Ingredient tip: This recipe also works well with other types of fish, such as tilapia or cod.

PER SERVING: Calories: 525; Total fat: 24g; Total carbohydrates: 38g; Fiber: 14g; Protein: 41g; Sodium: 223mg

Sardine Okonomiyaki

SERVES 4 / PREP TIME: 5 MINUTES / COOK TIME: 20 MINUTES

Sardines don't get a lot of attention. But they're a great source of healthy omega-3 fat. I prefer to call this dish by its Japanese name because "giant sardine pancake" isn't very appealing. My Peruvian Canadian sweetheart grew up in Lima eating these, but his mom divided the batter into small pancakes instead of one giant one. He knows them as *torrejas de sardinas*. Whatever you call them, it's worth stepping outside of your comfort zone and giving this recipe a try. It's delicious! A nonstick skillet works best for this recipe. If you have one, you can decrease the cooking oil to 2 tablespoons.

2 eggs

2 scallions, both white and green parts

1 cup flour

3 cups shredded cabbage (or coleslaw mix)

1 (4.4-ounce) can of sardines, drained

1 cup water

1 teaspoon reduced-sodium soy sauce

¼ cup vegetable oil

1. In a large bowl, beat the eggs.
2. Slice the scallions. Mix the scallion whites in with the eggs. Set the greens aside for later.
3. To the egg mixture, add the flour, cabbage, sardines, water, and soy sauce. Mix, mashing the sardines with your whisk.
4. Heat the oil in a large skillet over low-medium heat. Tip the okonomiyaki mixture into the pan and use a spatula to form it into a round pancake about ½-Inch thick. When golden brown on the bottom, carefully flip and cook the other side until it's golden, too.
5. Remove from the pan, divide the pancake in 4, and serve sprinkled with the scallion greens.

Cooking tip: If, like me, you're not good at flipping pancakes, I recommend using your spatula to cut the okonomiyaki into four pieces and flipping the pieces one at a time.

PER SERVING: Calories: 324; Total fat: 19g; Total carbohydrates: 26g; Fiber: 2g; Protein: 13g; Sodium: 220mg

8

VEGETARIAN/VEGAN MAINS

BLACK-EYED PEAS WITH KALE
AND SWEET POTATO, PAGE 149

Miso Soup with Tofu and Noodles

VEGETARIAN, VEGAN, GLUTEN-FREE

SERVES 4 / PREP TIME: 10 MINUTES / COOK TIME: 5 MINUTES

You likely know miso soup as an appetizer in sushi restaurants. This recipe transforms miso soup into a quick, light meal. There are different types of miso paste. Any of them will work in this recipe. I particularly like shiro or white miso for its more subtle flavor. You'll find tofu, miso paste, nori (roasted seaweed sheets), and enoki mushrooms in any supermarket with a good Asian food section. Omit the mushrooms if you can't find them. This is a really quick-cooking recipe, so take the time to prep your ingredients before adding anything to the water or stock.

½ cup miso paste

8½ cups water or vegetable stock

5 ounces rice stick or rice vermicelli noodles

1 (14-ounce) package of medium-firm or silken tofu, cut into ½-inch cubes

2 cups enoki mushrooms

1 sheet nori, cut into thin slices

4 cups spinach

½ cup scallions, sliced, for garnish (4 scallions)

4 teaspoons sesame seeds, for garnish

1. Put the miso paste in a small bowl. Set aside.

2. In a covered, large saucepan over medium heat, bring the water or stock to a simmer. When the water comes to a simmer, carefully remove ½ cup of liquid and add it to the miso paste. Stir to create a slurry.

3. Add the rice noodles to your saucepan. Cook the vermicelli noodles for 1 minute, stick noodles for 2 minutes. Add the miso slurry, tofu, mushrooms, and nori. Cook for 2 minutes. Take care not to boil the miso. Add the spinach, in batches if necessary. Cook for 1 minute.

4. Divide the soup into 4 serving bowls. Garnish with the scallions and sesame seeds. Serve immediately.

Equipment tip: Cut the nori into strips with a pair of sharp kitchen scissors.

PER SERVING: Calories: 244; Total fat: 6g; Total carbohydrates: 38g; Fiber: 3g; Protein: 11g; Sodium: 206mg

Black Bean Soup

VEGETARIAN, VEGAN (OPTION), GLUTEN-FREE, MAKES GREAT LEFTOVERS

SERVES 4 / PREP TIME: 5 MINUTES / COOK TIME: 15 MINUTES

This flavorful soup involves minimal prep and cooking time, making it a perfect dish for a rushed weeknight, such as Meatless Monday. Pair it with a piece of crusty whole grain bread to dip in the soup. I eat this in its vegan form, but you can garnish with sour cream, if you prefer. This recipe makes great leftovers. Store without the garnish in the refrigerator for 3 or 4 days, or in the freezer for 2 or 3 months.

1 tablespoon extra-virgin olive oil

1 yellow onion, diced

1 chile pepper, finely diced

2 green bell peppers, diced

1 garlic clove, minced

1 (28-ounce) can diced tomatoes

1 (15½-ounce) can black beans, drained and rinsed

3 cups water

1 teaspoon cumin

1 teaspoon chili powder

½ teaspoon ground black pepper

¼ teaspoon salt

Sour cream, for garnish (optional)

Fresh cilantro, chopped, for garnish (optional)

Hot sauce, for garnish (optional)

1. Heat the oil in a large saucepan over medium heat. Sauté the onion, stirring frequently for 2 minutes. Add the chile and bell peppers. Sauté, stirring, for 2 minutes. Add the garlic and continue to sauté, stirring, for 30 seconds.
2. Add the tomatoes, black beans, water, cumin, chili powder, pepper, and salt. Cover, increase the heat to high, and bring to a boil. Reduce the heat to medium and cook for 10 minutes.
3. To serve, divide among 4 serving bowls. Top with sour cream, fresh cilantro, and a dash of hot sauce if using.

Ingredient tip: Because tomatoes are technically a fruit, they contain some natural sugar, appearing as a few grams of sugar on the nutrition facts panel. This is not the free sugar that we're avoiding. Canned tomatoes are a fantastic pantry staple for creating many healthy dishes from scratch.

PER SERVING: Calories: 206; Total fat: 4g; Total carbohydrates: 36g; Fiber: 9g; Protein: 9g; Sodium: 611mg Sodium: 611mg

MAKE YOUR OWN (FREE) VEGETABLE STOCK

Did you know that you already have the ingredients to make the most delicious vegetable stock? That's right! And you've almost certainly been throwing them in the trash. Making your own vegetable stock is the secret to creating incredibly tasty vegetarian dishes, and it's free. All you use are the scraps from the vegetables that you're already buying. Here's how:

1. Put a resealable plastic bag in your freezer.
2. Every time that you have scraps from onions, leeks, shallots, carrots, and celery, put the scraps in your freezer bag. I'm talking about the parts that you usually throw away in your recycling bin, such as carrot peelings, the ends from celery stalks, the ends and outer skins from onions, and the green part of leeks.
3. When your freezer bag is full, put its contents into the largest saucepan that you own and fill it up with water.
4. Cover and bring it to a boil over high heat. Then lower the heat to low-medium and simmer, covered, for at least an hour.
5. Remove from the heat and allow to cool. Put a bowl underneath a colander. Strain the liquid. Put the scraps in your recycling bin.
6. Portion the golden liquid into reusable freezer containers. Freeze.
7. One day ahead of when you plan to make a recipe that calls for vegetable (or chicken) stock, pull out your frozen stock and defrost it in the refrigerator.

Vegetarian Borscht

VEGETARIAN, VEGAN (OPTION), GLUTEN-FREE, MAKES GREAT LEFTOVERS

SERVES 8 / PREP TIME: 15 MINUTES / COOK TIME: 1 HOUR 15 MINUTES

Beans, beets, and cabbage are all superfoods and inexpensive. As such, I'm always looking for new recipes that include them. Traditional borscht contains meat. This vegetarian borscht is a hearty and tasty one-pot meal. Serve it with a piece of crusty whole grain bread. While the recipe takes a bit longer to cook, it makes a lot of soup and makes great leftovers. Freeze the soup in small batches (without the dill and yogurt or sour cream garnish). It's especially handy to have healthy meals like this in the freezer during the busy holiday season.

3 tablespoons extra-virgin olive oil

1½ cups yellow onion, diced

2 garlic cloves, minced

2 cups diced carrots

1 cup diced celery

4 cups green cabbage, shredded

3 cups beets, peeled and chopped into ½-inch pieces

10 cups vegetable stock

2 (15½-ounce) cans cannellini beans, drained and rinsed

½ cup canned, diced tomatoes

½ cup tomato juice

2 tablespoons lemon juice

1 teaspoon ground black pepper

½ teaspoon salt

4 tablespoons fresh dill, chopped, for garnish

½ cup plain yogurt or sour cream, for garnish (optional)

1. Heat the oil in your largest saucepan over medium heat. Add the onions and sauté, stirring, for 2 minutes. Add the garlic and sauté for 30 seconds. Add the carrots, celery, and cabbage and sauté, stirring, for 3 minutes.
2. Add the beets and stock and cook, covered for 1 hour, stirring occasionally
3. Add the beans, tomatoes, tomato juice, lemon juice, pepper, and salt. Warm thoroughly, about 5 minutes.
4. To serve, divide the soup among 8 serving bowls. Top each bowl with fresh dill and a dollop of yogurt or sour cream, if using.

Ingredient tip: This is a perfect recipe for homemade vegetable stock (page 138).

PER SERVING: Calories: 241; Total fat: 6g; Total carbohydrates: 36g; Fiber: 9g; Protein: 12g; Sodium: 1005mg

Pineapple Peanut Stew

VEGETARIAN, VEGAN, GLUTEN-FREE, MAKE AHEAD

SERVES 4 / PREP TIME: 5 MINUTES / COOK TIME: 20 MINUTES

This is a unique stew. It's sweet and salty like a peanut butter and jelly sandwich but in a whole different way. I prefer crunchy peanut butter for this recipe, but smooth will work as well. Serve it with brown rice to complete the meal. It's very quick to make, so it's a fantastic recipe for rushed weekday dinners. The strong flavors of the peanut butter and pineapple overpower the bitterness of the kale, so it's a great recipe for fledgling kale eaters.

1 tablespoon vegetable oil

½ cup yellow onion, diced (½ onion)

1 orange bell pepper, diced

1 chile pepper, minced

1 garlic clove, minced

1 cup fresh pineapple, diced

1 cup water

½ teaspoon salt

½ teaspoon ground black pepper

8 cups kale, chopped

½ cup natural peanut butter

1 cup peanuts

4 cups cooked brown rice

1. Heat the oil in a large saucepan over medium heat. Add the onions and sauté, stirring, for 2 minutes. Add the bell pepper and chile pepper. Sauté, stirring for 1 minute. Add the garlic. Sauté, stirring for 1 minute.

2. Add the pineapple, water, salt, and pepper. Bring to a boil. Add the kale in batches. Sauté, stirring for 3 minutes, until the kale is just wilted.

3. Stir in the peanut butter. Cook for 5 minutes, stirring constantly. Add in the peanuts for the final minute of cooking.

4. To serve, divide the rice among 4 serving bowls. Top with the stew. Serve immediately.

Ingredient tip: Most of the heat in a chile pepper is found in the internal white membrane and the seeds. If you can't handle the heat, remove all, or some, of this membrane and seeds to get some chile flavor without much heat.

PER SERVING: Calories: 768; Total fat: 41g; Total carbohydrates: 85g; Fiber: 16g; Protein: 28g; Sodium: 357mg

Eggplant and Chickpea Stew

VEGETARIAN, VEGAN, GLUTEN-FREE, MAKE AHEAD

SERVES 4 / PREP TIME: 10 MINUTES / COOK TIME: 25 MINUTES

Many people say that they don't like eggplant, but that's probably just because they haven't had it cooked properly. The key step to cooking eggplant is salting it to bring out the bitterness, then rinsing it away. For this recipe, you want the Mediterranean-style, bulbous eggplant, not the long, skinny, Asian style. Serve this dish with brown rice or Saffron Quinoa (page 179).

1 eggplant

2 teaspoons salt, divided

3 tablespoons extra-virgin olive oil

1 cup finely diced yellow onion (1 onion)

2 green bell peppers, cut into 1-inch pieces

2 garlic cloves, minced

1 chile pepper, finely diced

2 (15½-ounce) cans chickpeas, drained and rinsed

1 (28-ounce) can diced tomatoes

1 cup water

1 tablespoon dried oregano

1 bay leaf

2 teaspoons dried basil

1 teaspoon ground black pepper

4 cups cooked quinoa or brown rice

1. Remove the stem from the eggplant. Cut it into 1-inch cubes. Sprinkle a large plate with 1 teaspoon of salt. Place the eggplant on the plate in an even layer. Sprinkle with the remaining teaspoon of salt. Set it aside.

2. Heat the oil in a large saucepan over medium heat. Add the onion and sauté, stirring, for 3 minutes. Add the bell peppers, garlic, and chile pepper. Sauté for 1 minute.

3. In a colander, rinse the eggplant. Add it to the saucepan, and sauté for 1 minute.

4. Add the chickpeas, tomatoes, water, oregano, bay leaf, basil, and pepper. Cover, increase the heat to high, and bring the stew to a boil. Lower the heat to medium and cook, stirring occasionally, until the eggplant is cooked through, about 20 minutes.

5. To serve, divide among 4 serving bowls, on top of 1 cup of quinoa or brown rice.

Storage tip: If you're not cooking for 4, this makes great leftovers. Store in the refrigerator for 3 or 4 days or in the freezer for 2 or 3 months.

PER SERVING: Calories: 672; Total fat: 19g; Total carbohydrates: 104g; Fiber: 24g; Protein: 25g; Sodium: 1,578mg

Coconut Red Lentils

VEGETARIAN, VEGAN, GLUTEN-FREE

SERVES 4 / PREP TIME: 5 MINUTES / COOK TIME: 20 MINUTES

Red lentils are the quickest cooking of any bean and lentil. Even better, they don't need to be soaked before cooking. So, they're perfect for a busy weeknight. This dish is satisfying and warming on a dark, dreary evening—in other words, just about every night between November and March here on the rainy West Coast. I like this dish served with brown rice or Spiced Rice and Peas (page 182) and simple steamed green veggies, such as green beans or broccoli.

4 cups water

1¼ cups red lentils

¼ teaspoon turmeric

1 tablespoon grated ginger

1 chile pepper, whole

¼ teaspoon salt

¼ teaspoon ground black pepper

¼ cup coconut milk, stirred to mix the thin and thick parts before measuring

2 tablespoons lime juice

4 cups cooked rice

1. Bring the water to a boil in a large saucepan over high heat. Add the red lentils and return to a boil, then lower the heat to low-medium. With a spoon, remove and discard any foam from the top. Add the turmeric, ginger, chile pepper, salt, and pepper. Simmer, covered, until the lentils are very soft, about 15 minutes.

2. Remove from the heat and discard the chile pepper.

3. Purée the mixture in a blender until smooth. An immersion blender is perfect for this step. Stir in the coconut milk and warm over low heat, continuously stirring, about 5 minutes. Remove from the heat and stir in the lime juice.

4. To serve, divide rice among 4 serving dishes. Top with the lentils.

Storage tip: This dish doesn't make great leftovers. If you're not cooking for four people, divide the recipe in half but still use one whole chile pepper.

PER SERVING: Calories: 439; Total fat: 6g; Total carbohydrates: 78g; Fiber: 20g; Protein: 20g; Sodium: 161mg

North African Chickpea Stew

VEGETARIAN, VEGAN, GLUTEN-FREE, MAKES GREAT LEFTOVERS

SERVES 4 / PREP TIME: 5 MINUTES / COOK TIME: 10 MINUTES

The traditional flavors of the Mediterranean and North Africa come together in this unusual stew. I call it unusual because you likely recognize all of the ingredients; however, when combined in this recipe, the stew has a unique and delicious flavor. This is an excellent recipe for those who are new to eating kale. All of the strong flavors in the stew mask kale's bitter taste. Don't be concerned with the couple of grams of sugar that you see in the nutrition facts panel on tomato juice and tomato paste. That's the natural sugar found within tomatoes. Check the ingredient lists to make sure there isn't any added free sugar.

1 tablespoon extra-virgin olive oil

1 cup diced yellow onion (1 onion)

4 cups kale, middle strip removed and coarsely chopped

1 garlic clove, minced

2 teaspoons ground coriander

½ teaspoon turmeric

½ teaspoon salt

¼ teaspoon cayenne

⅛ teaspoon cinnamon

4 cups water

2 (15½-ounce) cans chickpeas, drained and rinsed

1 (12-ounce) jar roasted red peppers, rinsed

½ cup slivered almonds

1 cup tomato juice

1 (6-ounce) can tomato paste

¼ cup raisins

¼ cup dried apricots, diced

1 tablespoon lemon juice

1. Heat the oil in a large saucepan over medium heat. Add the onions and sauté, stirring, for 2 minutes. Add the kale, garlic, coriander, turmeric, salt, cayenne, and cinnamon. Sauté for 1 minute.

2. Add the water, chickpeas, red peppers, slivered almonds, tomato juice, tomato paste, raisins, and apricots. Cover and bring to a boil over high heat. Reduce the heat to low-medium and simmer for 5 minutes, stirring occasionally.

3. Stir in the lemon juice immediately before serving. To serve, divide the stew among 4 serving bowls.

Storage tip: The flavors continue to mingle as the stew sits, so it makes great leftovers. Store in the refrigerator for 3 or 4 days. Store in the freezer for 2 or 3 months.

PER SERVING: Calories: 527; Total fat: 15g; Total carbohydrates: 85g; Fiber: 22g; Protein: 23g; Sodium: 843mg

Warm Potato Salad with Hard-Boiled Eggs and Green Beans

VEGETARIAN, GLUTEN-FREE, MAKE AHEAD (OPTION)

SERVES 4 / PREP TIME: 10 MINUTES / COOK TIME: 20 MINUTES

This is a perfect dinner on a hot summer evening when you want a light meal. It celebrates fresh, in-season new potatoes and green beans. It's unfussy yet elegant—perfect for casual summer dinner parties on the patio. Serve on its own or with some sliced in-season tomatoes on the side. Finish the meal with a light, refreshing dessert such as Cantaloupe Granita (page 188).

FOR THE SALAD

8 hard-boiled eggs

4 cups new potatoes

8 cups green beans, ends removed and beans snapped in half

FOR THE DRESSING

¼ cup extra-virgin olive oil

1 shallot, finely diced

1 garlic clove, minced

¼ cup balsamic vinegar

1 teaspoon salt

1 teaspoon ground black pepper

1. Follow the directions on page 35 to hard-boil the eggs.
2. Bring your largest saucepan of water to a boil over high heat.
3. Prepare the potatoes. Leave smaller new potatoes whole. Cut larger ones in half or quarters, so that all of your potatoes are about the same size. When the water boils, add the potatoes. Boil for 12 minutes. Add the green beans and boil for another 3 minutes. Drain the potatoes and beans using a colander and put the veggies in a serving dish. With a fork, smash the whole potatoes to expose the flesh before pouring on the dressing.
4. While the potatoes are boiling, prepare the dressing. Heat the oil in a small saucepan over medium heat. Add the shallots and garlic. Sauté 3 minutes, until the shallots are translucent. Remove from the heat. Add the balsamic vinegar, salt, and pepper. Stir to combine. Set aside.
5. Peel the hard-boiled eggs and cut into quarters. Arrange around the potatoes and beans.

6. Add the dressing to the potatoes and eggs, and serve immediately.

Make ahead tip: Cook the hard-boiled eggs ahead of time to make this dish even easier to prepare.

PER SERVING: Calories: 464; Total fat: 24g; Total carbohydrates: 46g; Fiber: 9g; Protein: 20g; Sodium: 724mg

Tofu and Pea Curry

VEGETARIAN, VEGAN, GLUTEN-FREE, MAKE AHEAD, MAKES GREAT LEFTOVERS

SERVES 4 / PREP TIME: 15 MINUTES / COOK TIME: 20 MINUTES

I thought curry involved hundreds of complicated steps and ingredients. Then I learned I was wrong. Once you see how easy it is to make your own spice paste, you won't be dialing for takeout anymore.

FOR THE SPICE PASTE

3 tomatoes, coarsely chopped

½ cup onion, coarsely chopped

2 garlic cloves

1 chile pepper

1-by-1-inch piece of fresh ginger

¼ cup cashews

½ teaspoon ground black pepper

½ teaspoon ground coriander

¼ teaspoon ground cloves

¼ teaspoon cinnamon

FOR THE CURRY

2 tablespoons vegetable oil

½ teaspoon cumin seeds

¼ teaspoon turmeric

½ teaspoon garam masala powder

¼ teaspoon salt

4 cups frozen peas

1 (14-ounce) package firm or extra-firm tofu, cut into ½-inch cubes

4 cups cooked brown rice

1. Combine all of the ingredients for the spice paste in a blender. Put the tomatoes in first to provide the liquid to get it blending. Purée until smooth. Set aside.

2. Heat the oil in a large skillet over medium heat. Sauté the cumin seeds for 15 seconds, until fragrant. Add the spice paste. Sauté, stirring frequently, for 5 minutes. Add the turmeric, garam masala, and salt and cook, stirring, for 3 more minutes. Add the peas, and tofu, and cook, stirring frequently, for 10 minutes.

3. To serve, divide the rice among 4 serving bowls. Top with the curry.

Ingredient tip: To make this curry extra creamy, add 1 tablespoon of cream along with the peas and tofu in step 2. Keep in mind that this will make the recipe no longer vegan.

PER SERVING: Calories: 578; Total fat: 19g; Total carbohydrates: 80g; Fiber: 13g; Protein: 25g; Sodium: 376mg

Smokey Tempeh

VEGETARIAN, VEGAN, GLUTEN-FREE (OPTION), MAKE AHEAD

SERVES 4 / PREP TIME: 5 MINUTES / COOK TIME: 5 MINUTES

Yes, this dinner really is ready in 10 minutes. Tempeh is a fermented soy product, similar to tofu, but made using a different method. Like tofu, it is a good source of protein. But unlike blank-slate tofu, tempeh has an earthy flavor. In this recipe, that earthy flavor is played up to create a deep smokiness flavor, reminiscent of barbequed meat. Serve your tempeh with Build Your Own Slaw (page 169) and leftover brown rice to round out your 10-minute meal.

½ **cup reduced-sodium soy sauce (or gluten-free tamari, if desired)**

¼ **cup balsamic vinegar**

¼ **cup extra-virgin olive oil**

2 **garlic cloves**

¾ **teaspoon ground black pepper**

2 **(8-ounce) packages tempeh**

1. In a medium bowl, combine the soy sauce, balsamic vinegar, oil, garlic, and pepper.
2. Cut the tempeh into 1 ½-inch cubes. Add it to the marinade. Toss to coat every side of the tempeh pieces in marinade.
3. In a large skillet over low-medium heat, sauté for 5 minutes. Flip halfway through cooking. To serve, divide the tempeh among 4 serving plates with your sides.

Make ahead tip: You can make this a 5-minute meal by doing your prep in the morning. Combine the marinade ingredients and add the tempeh. Cover and refrigerate. Then, when you get home in the evening, heat up your skillet and cook.

PER SERVING: Calories: 390; Total fat: 24g; Total carbohydrates: 20g; Fiber: 9g; Protein: 22g; Sodium: 1,165mg

Caribbean Tofu

VEGETARIAN, VEGAN, GLUTEN-FREE, MAKES GREAT LEFTOVERS

SERVES 4 / PREP TIME: 10 MINUTES / COOK TIME: 5 MINUTES

You won't believe how quick this recipe is to make—or, how delicious it tastes. There's nowhere for this tofu to hide, so it's not for the beginner tofu eater. This dish celebrates tofu for those of us who love it. In this recipe, we take it on a Caribbean vacation. I love this dish in the summertime, paired with a tossed salad or slaw and Saffron Quinoa (page 179).

2 garlic cloves

¼ cup lime juice

¼ cup fresh cilantro, chopped

¼ cup vegetable oil

1 tablespoon orange zest (1 orange)

1 teaspoon cumin

¼ teaspoon salt

¼ teaspoon pepper

1 (14-ounce) package firm or extra-firm tofu

1. In a medium bowl, combine the garlic, lime juice, cilantro, vegetable oil, orange zest, cumin, salt, and pepper.
2. Cut the tofu into 1-inch cubes. Add it to the marinade. Toss to coat.
3. Pour the tofu and marinade into a large skillet over medium heat. Sauté, stirring, until the tofu is heated through and browning on the edges, about 5 minutes. To serve, divide the tofu among 4 serving plates with your sides.

Storage tip: This tofu, served cold, makes a delicious ingredient in a salad bowl. Or, eat it alongside some sliced orange bell pepper for an afternoon snack. Store leftover tofu in a resealable container in the refrigerator for 3 or 4 days. It does not freeze well.

PER SERVING: Calories: 224; Total fat: 18g; Total carbohydrates: 6g; Fiber: 2g; Protein: 11g; Sodium: 163mg

Black-Eyed Peas with Kale and Sweet Potato

VEGETARIAN, VEGAN, GLUTEN-FREE, MAKES GREAT LEFTOVERS

SERVES 4 / PREP TIME: 10 MINUTES / COOK TIME: 20 MINUTES

It's amazing how a few ingredients can make a complete dish. This is great meal for a rushed weeknight. It's also a good introduction to kale, because the sweetness from the yams and the apple cider vinegar counteract kale's bitterness. This dish also makes great leftovers. I particularly like this dish served cold for lunch in the summertime, because it's like a cross between a good bean salad and a potato salad.

2 cups yams, peeled and cut in ½-inch pieces

1 tablespoon extra-virgin olive oil

1 cup diced yellow onion (1 onion)

1 chile pepper, minced

1 garlic clove, minced

6 cups kale, coarsely chopped and middle stems removed

2 (15½-ounce) cans black-eyed peas, drained and rinsed

1 tablespoon apple cider vinegar

¼ teaspoon salt

¼ teaspoon ground black pepper

1. Cook the yam in a large saucepan of boiling water until tender, about 10 minutes.
2. Heat the oil in a large skillet over low-medium heat. Add the onions and sauté, stirring, for 4 minutes. Add the chile pepper and sauté, stirring, for 2 minutes. Add the garlic and sauté, stirring, for 30 seconds. Add the kale and sauté, stirring, for 2 minutes. Add the black-eyed peas, cooked yams, vinegar, salt, and pepper. Sauté, stirring, for 2 minutes. To serve, divide the peas mixture among 4 serving bowls.

Ingredient tip: This recipe calls for about 3½ cups of black-eyed peas. If using peas prepared from scratch, soak just under 1¾ cups of raw peas to make 3½ cups cooked peas. This dish also works with black beans and pinto beans. Cannellini and white navy beans can work in a pinch.

PER SERVING: Calories: 359; Total fat: 6g; Total carbohydrates: 64g; Fiber: 14g; Protein: 14g; Sodium: 205mg

Vegetable Frittata

VEGETARIAN, GLUTEN-FREE

SERVES 4 / PREP TIME: 15 MINUTES / COOK TIME: 30 MINUTES, PLUS 5 MINUTES TO REST

I love this frittata recipe. Who doesn't love breakfast for dinner? And it is so versatile. I've used all sorts of veggie combos. I particularly like this recipe in the spring when the nettles are growing wild and the local asparagus comes into season. You may not be able to go foraging for stinging nettles, so here I've used universally available (and delicious) Swiss chard and mushrooms. This is a veggie-heavy frittata. The veggies make up the body of your dish, with the egg holding everything together. Serve with a tossed salad and piece of whole grain bread.

Cooking oil spray

5 eggs

¼ cup milk

1 teaspoon powdered mustard

½ teaspoon salt

1 tablespoon extra-virgin olive oil

½ cup diced yellow onion (½ onion)

1 garlic clove, minced

1½ cups mushrooms, sliced

4 cups Swiss chard, chopped

⅓ cup shredded cheddar cheese

½ cup fresh parsley, chopped, for garnish

1. Preheat the oven to 375°F.
2. Coat a 9-inch glass pie plate with cooking oil spray. Set aside.
3. In a medium bowl, beat together the eggs, milk, mustard, and salt. Set aside.
4. Heat the oil in a large skillet over medium heat. Add the onions and sauté, stirring, for 2 minutes. Add the garlic and sauté for 30 seconds. Add the mushrooms and sauté, stirring, for 2 minutes. Add the Swiss chard in batches. Sauté, stirring, until just wilted, about 3 minutes.
5. Transfer veggies to the pie plate. Pour in the egg mixture and top with the shredded cheese.
6. Bake in the oven until the center is golden brown, about 20 to 25 minutes. Let the frittata rest 5 minutes before serving. To serve, cut your frittata in 4 pieces and garnish with parsley. Put one piece on each of 4 serving plates next to your salad and bread.

Storage tip: This recipe makes great leftovers. Store in the refrigerator for 3 or 4 days. Serve warm or cold. It doesn't freeze well.

PER SERVING: Calories: 215; Total fat: 13g; Total carbohydrates: 12g; Fiber: 5g; Protein: 15g; Sodium: 761mg

Black Bean Stir-Fry

VEGETARIAN, VEGAN, GLUTEN-FREE (OPTION), MAKE AHEAD

SERVES 4 / PREP TIME: 15 MINUTES / COOK TIME: 5 MINUTES

Don't you love how fast stir-fries are to cook? It makes them the quintessential quick dish for rushed weeknight dinners. This is a great dish for a fledgling vegan or those new to plant-based eating. The mushrooms provide the umami flavor that meat provides in a dish. Mix and match the veggies as you want, but do keep the mushrooms. For example, kale, celery, water chestnuts, and baby corn are all fantastic in this recipe. Serve it over brown rice to complete your meal.

1 tablespoon sesame oil

1 tablespoon vegetable oil

¼ cup reduced-sodium soy sauce (or gluten-free tamari, if desired)

2 tablespoon rice vinegar

1 teaspoon red chili flakes

1 red bell pepper, sliced

2 cups mushrooms, sliced

2 cups snow peas, ends and strings removed

2 cups bok choy, coarsely chopped

1 yellow onion, thinly sliced

2 garlic clove, minced

2-by-1-inch piece of fresh ginger, minced

1 (15½-ounce) can black beans, drained and rinsed

4 cups brown rice

1. Heat the sesame and vegetable oils in a large skillet over medium-high heat.

2. In a small bowl, combine the soy sauce, vinegar, and red chili flakes.

3. Add the bell pepper, mushrooms, snow peas, bok choy, onion, garlic, ginger, and black beans to your pan, in batches if necessary. If you need to do batches, include mushrooms in the first batch and leafy greens (e.g., bok choy) in the last batch. Stir the entire time. Cook 4 minutes. Pour in the sauce and cook for more minute.

4. To serve, divide the rice among 4 serving bowls. Top with the stir-fry.

Ingredient tip: Reduce your prep time by leaving the snow peas whole. I find the tougher strings unpleasant, so I take the time to remove them.

PER SERVING: Calories: 435; Total fat: 9g; Total carbohydrates: 74g; Fiber: 11g; Protein: 15g; Sodium: 604mg

Edamame Fried Rice

VEGETARIAN, GLUTEN-FREE (OPTION), MAKE AHEAD

SERVES 4 / PREP TIME: 10 MINUTES / COOK TIME: 10 MINUTES

Who doesn't love fried rice? If you have a wok, use it for this dish. Mix and match the vegetables. For example, bok choy, kale, and the stems from Swiss chard would all work well. Do keep the mushrooms in the dish, as they provide the umami flavor necessary for a good fried rice.

1½ cups edamame, frozen

2 eggs

2 tablespoons sesame oil

3 cups mushrooms, sliced

1½ cups carrots, sliced

1 cup sliced celery

½ cup sliced scallions (about 4 scallions), whites separated from the greens

2 garlic cloves, minced

1-by-1-inch piece fresh ginger, minced

1 teaspoon ground black pepper

3 cups leftover brown rice

¼ cup reduced-sodium soy sauce (or gluten-free tamari, if desired)

2 cups bean sprouts

1. Take the edamame out of the freezer while you prepare the remaining ingredients.

2. Break the eggs into a small bowl. Set aside.

3. Heat the oil in a large skillet over medium heat. Add the mushrooms, carrots, celery, white part of scallions, garlic, ginger, edamame, and black pepper. Sauté 3 minutes, stirring. Add the rice and sauté for 2 more minutes, stirring. Add the egg and soy sauce. Sauté 2 minutes, then add the bean sprouts. Sauté 1 minute.

4. Garnish with the green part of the scallions and a drizzle of sesame oil. Serve immediately, adding extra soy sauce, if desired.

Ingredient tip: You can find edamame in the frozen vegetables section of any supermarket that carries Asian foods. Edamame in its pods makes a great snack (simply cook in boiling water for 5 minutes, then sprinkle with salt). This recipe uses edamame without the pods.

PER SERVING: Calories: 386; Total fat: 13g; Total carbohydrates: 50g; Fiber: 6g; Protein: 18g; Sodium: 726mg

Tomato-Ricotta Spaghetti

VEGETARIAN, GLUTEN-FREE (OPTION)

SERVES 4 / PREP TIME: 5 MINUTES / COOK TIME: 20 MINUTES

I was taught this recipe a lifetime ago when an Italian houseguest visited my roommate. She also taught me that good pasta is all about a few beautiful ingredients. Don't try this recipe with watery, pale tomatoes. You need full-flavor tomatoes, extra-virgin olive oil, and ideally, fresh ground black pepper. This recipe doesn't make good leftovers. If cooking for two people, divide the recipe in half and use 1 or 2 cloves of garlic, depending on how garlicky you like your food.

12 ounces whole wheat spaghetti noodles (gluten-free, if desired)

2 tablespoons extra-virgin olive oil

3 garlic cloves, minced

4 cups cherry or grape tomatoes, halved

½ teaspoon salt

½ teaspoon ground black pepper

2 cups ricotta cheese

1. Bring a large pot of water to a boil over high heat. Add the pasta and cook until al dente, 5 to 8 minutes, depending on the shape of the pasta.
2. Heat the oil in a large skillet over medium heat. Add the garlic and sauté, stirring, for 30 seconds. Add the tomatoes and continue to sauté, stirring, for 5 minutes.
3. Add the salt and pepper, and stir in the ricotta. Cook for 2 minutes, continuously stirring until the ricotta has melted into the tomatoes.
4. Divide the pasta among 4 serving dishes and serve immediately.

Ingredient tip: Up the vegetable quotient of this recipe by adding 4 cups of spinach, sautéed for 1 minute before adding the ricotta.

PER SERVING: Calories: 549; Total fat: 19g; Total carbohydrates: 63g; Fiber: 8g; Protein: 27g; Sodium: 488mg

Beans and Greens Pesto Pasta

VEGETARIAN, VEGAN (OPTION), GLUTEN-FREE (OPTION)

SERVES 4 / PREP TIME: 10 MINUTES / COOK TIME: 15 MINUTES

This is my go-to meal when I need dinner FAST. I probably eat it once a week. What's even better is that it involves not just one, but two superfoods: leafy greens and beans. You likely already know that leafy greens are chock-full of vitamins and minerals. Beans are a fantastic source of vegetarian protein and fiber. Feel free to change up your beans and leafy greens. For example, Romano beans work well instead of the cannellini beans. Spinach and baby kale work in place of the Swiss chard.

12 ounces whole wheat pasta noodles of your choice (gluten-free, if desired)

1 tablespoon extra-virgin olive oil

½ cup diced yellow onion (½ onion)

2 garlic cloves, minced

8 cups Swiss chard, coarsely chopped, stemmed (save them for another dish)

1 (15½ ounce) can cannellini beans, drained and rinsed

4 tablespoons pesto (dairy-free if desired)

Parmesan cheese, for garnish (optional)

1. In a large saucepan of boiling water, cook the noodles until al dente, about 6 to 8 minutes.
2. Heat the oil in a large skillet over medium heat. Add the onions and sauté, stirring, for 2 minutes. Add the garlic and sauté for 30 seconds. Add the chard (in batches, if necessary), beans, and pesto. Cook, stirring often, just until the greens wilt, about 3 minutes
3. Drain the cooked pasta and add it to the skillet with your greens. Thoroughly mix the noodles in with the sauce.
4. Divide the pasta among 4 serving dishes and sprinkle with Parmesan cheese, if using.

Storage tip: This dish makes a delicious cold pasta salad. Make extra and enjoy the leftovers for lunch or a picnic the following day.

PER SERVING: Calories: 554; Total fat: 12g; Total carbohydrates: 84g; Fiber: 18g; Protein: 26g; Sodium: 867mg

HOW TO COOK BEANS FROM SCRATCH

Beans, lentils, split peas, and chickpeas, when cooked from scratch (i.e., dry), are only pennies per serving. That's why they are a staple in my house. Twice a week or so, I cook up a big batch and use them in all sorts of dishes. Here's how to cook dry pulses without any fancy equipment.

1. **Soak overnight. Beans and chickpeas need to be soaked overnight to shorten the cooking time and to make them easier to digest (less gassy). Lentils don't need to be soaked overnight. Put your beans in a bowl and cover with enough water to come up 2 inches above the surface of your beans. Leave on the counter overnight (i.e., don't refrigerate). My mom always covered the bowl with a tea towel, so I do too.**

2. **Drain and rinse. Using a colander or sieve, drain your beans. Then rinse them under running water to remove any remaining soaking liquid.**

3. **Cook. Put your beans in a large saucepan. Add 3 parts water to 1 part beans. For example, if you measured out 1 cup of dried beans to soak, use 3 cups of water. Cover and bring to a boil over high heat. Remove the lid, lower to low-medium heat, and skim off any foam that has been created. Replace the lid and cook until the beans are soft. The length of your cooking time will depend on the size of the lentil or bean. For example, lentils take 20 to 25 minutes, black beans take 60 to 90 minutes, and chickpeas take 90 minutes to 2 hours. Drain the beans and store in the refrigerator for up to 1 week or in the freezer for up to 3 months.**

White Bean and Pumpkin Pasta

VEGETARIAN, VEGAN, GLUTEN-FREE (OPTION)

SERVES 4 / PREP TIME: 5 MINUTES / COOK TIME: 15 MINUTES

This fall-inspired recipe is both super easy and a great way to sneak in beans for those new to plant-based eating. Its sweeter flavor profile works for (picky) kids. I know that pumpkin, coconut, and pasta sound like a strange combination, but this dish really does taste great. It's also very quick to prepare, making this a perfect Meatless Monday meal.

12 ounces whole wheat linguine (gluten-free, if desired)

1 (15½-ounce) can white beans, drained and rinsed

1 (15½-ounce) can pumpkin purée

1 cup coconut milk

1 tablespoon extra-virgin olive oil

1 cup spinach, cut into ribbons

3 garlic cloves, minced

Vegetable stock (optional)

1. In a large saucepan of boiling water, cook the noodles until al dente, about 6 to 8 minutes.
2. Combine the beans, pumpkin, and coconut milk in a blender. Purée until smooth. Be patient, this can take a little while.
3. Heat the oil in a large skillet over medium heat. Sauté the spinach ribbons until wilted, about 1 or 2 minutes. Remove the spinach ribbons from the pan and set aside.
4. To the same oil, add the minced garlic and sauté, stirring, for 30 seconds. Add the pumpkin mixture to the garlic. Bring to a boil, stirring. Reduce the heat and simmer for a few minutes, stirring occasionally. If the sauce appears thick, add the vegetable stock or water 1 tablespoon at a time.
5. Add the cooked pasta to the skillet and mix.
6. Divide the pasta among 4 serving dishes and top with the spinach ribbons.

Storage tip: This recipe doesn't store well, so only cook as much as you need for dinner tonight. The recipe is easily divided in half using 1 or 2 cloves of garlic, depending on how much garlic you enjoy.

PER SERVING: Calories: 551; Total fat: 16g; Total carbohydrates: 76g; Fiber: 15g; Protein: 21g; Sodium: 66mg

J-K's Spaghetti

VEGETARIAN, VEGAN, GLUTEN-FREE (OPTION), MAKES GREAT LEFTOVERS

PASTA SERVES 4 / SAUCE SERVES 8 / PREP TIME: 10 MINUTES / COOK TIME: 1 HOUR 15 MINUTES

I grew up eating a beef version of this recipe. Here, I've adapted my mom's recipe to make it vegan. The J is for Jenefer (my mom) and the K is for Kristen (me). While this recipe does take a long time to cook, it makes a big batch of sauce. The sauce improves with time, so put some in the freezer in single-meal containers for quick dinners on busy weeknights. If you only want to cook enough sauce for 4 people, simply divide the recipe in half and serve with the full 12 ounces of pasta noodles.

2 tablespoons extra-virgin olive oil

1 onion, diced

2 garlic cloves, minced

1 chile pepper (e.g, jalapeño), finely chopped

2 cups chopped green bell pepper

1 cup chopped red bell pepper

1 (28-ounce) can diced tomatoes

1 (6-ounce) can tomato paste

⅓ cup red wine

2 bay leaves

1 tablespoon dried oregano

2 tablespoons dried parsley

1 teaspoon salt

1 teaspoon ground black pepper

1 pound veggie (tofu) ground round

12 ounces whole wheat spaghetti noodles (gluten-free, if desired)

1. Heat the oil in your largest saucepan, over low-medium heat. Add the onion and sauté, stirring, for 4 minutes. Add the garlic and chile pepper. Sauté, stirring, for 30 more seconds.
2. Add the bell peppers and sauté, stirring, for 4 minutes.
3. Add tomatoes, tomato paste, wine, bay leaves, oregano, parsley, salt, and pepper.
4. Cook the sauce, uncovered, for at least an hour, stirring occasionally. The longer you cook the sauce, the better the flavor. Add the veggie ground round in the final 10 minutes of cooking.
5. In a large saucepan of boiling water, cook the noodles until al dente, about 6 to 8 minutes. Drain the noodles using a colander.
6. Divide the cooked noodles among 4 serving plates. Top with the pasta sauce.

Ingredient tip: Unlike ground meat, veggie ground round is already cooked, so you want to add it at the end of cooking to warm it through.

PER SERVING: Calories: 450; Total fat: 6g; Total carbohydrates: 68g; Fiber: 11g; Protein: 25g; Sodium: 954mg

Spinach and Orzo Pie

VEGETARIAN

SERVES 4 / PREP TIME: 30 MINUTES / COOK TIME: 45 MINUTES

This meal is pure comfort food. I mean, you've got three kinds of cheese pairing up with pasta. That's basically the definition of comfort food, isn't it? Since this recipe also contains leafy greens, it's dietitian-approved comfort food. Use canned tomato sauce and not canned pasta sauce. Pasta sauce usually has free sugar added.

1½ cups orzo

2 large eggs

1 (15½-ounce) can of tomato sauce, divided

⅓ cup grated Parmesan cheese

Cooking oil spray

1 (10-ounce) package frozen, chopped spinach

½ cup ricotta cheese

¼ teaspoon nutmeg

½ cup shredded part-skim mozzarella cheese

1. Preheat the oven to 350°F.
2. In a large saucepan of boiling water, cook the orzo until al dente, about 6 to 8 minutes.
3. Beat the eggs in a medium bowl. Add ½ cup of the tomato sauce, Parmesan, and the cooked orzo. Stir to combine.
4. Coat a 9-inch glass pie plate (bottom and sides) with cooking oil spray. Spread the orzo mixture over the bottom and up the sides of the pie plate to form a crust.
5. In a microwave on medium, cook the spinach until just warm, about 4 minutes. Drain well by pressing it in a colander to squeeze out the liquid.
6. In a medium bowl, add the spinach, ricotta, and nutmeg. Stir to thoroughly combine. Spoon the mixture into the pie plate.
7. Spread the remaining tomato sauce over the spinach mixture. Cover the orzo crust with foil.
8. Bake for 30 minutes. Remove the foil and sprinkle with the mozzarella. Return to the oven and bake the pie until the mozzarella is melted and bubbling, about 3 to 5 minutes.
9. Let the pie rest for 5 minutes before serving. To serve, cut the pie into 4 pieces.

PER SERVING: Calories: 463; Total fat: 11g; Total carbohydrates: 63g; Fiber: 7g; Protein: 27g; Sodium: 952mg

Pinto Bean Pie

VEGETARIAN, GLUTEN-FREE (OPTION)

SERVES 4 / PREP TIME: 15 MINUTES / COOK TIME: 1 HOUR

I guess that savory pies must have had a moment back in the 1980s, because, similar to Spinach and Orzo Pie (page 158), I remember this dish from my childhood. While these savory pies do take a bit more effort to prepare, they are very approachable dishes for those new to plant-based eating. In this dish, the classic flavors of Mexican cuisine are combined and topped with a cornmeal crust that bakes up golden brown, reminiscent of corn bread.

2½ cups water

½ cup extra-virgin olive oil

1½ cups cornmeal

1 cup all-purpose flour (gluten-free, if desired)

1 teaspoon cumin

½ teaspoon salt, divided

1 (15½-ounce) can pinto beans

1 (15-ounce) can tomato sauce

1 green bell pepper, diced

1 chile pepper, finely diced

2 garlic cloves

¼ teaspoon salt

1 teaspoon dried oregano

Cooking oil spray

1. Preheat the oven to 325°F.

2. In a large bowl, combine the water, olive oil, cornmeal, flour, cumin, and ¼ teaspoon salt. Stir well to combine. Set aside.

3. Drain and rinse the beans. In a second large bowl, combine the beans, tomato sauce, bell pepper, chile pepper, garlic, salt, and oregano.

4. Coat a 9-inch glass pie plate (bottom and sides) with the cooking oil spray. Pour in half of the cornmeal mixture. Pour the bean mixture on top of the cornmeal, and top with the second half of the cornmeal mixture.

5. Bake until the cornmeal is set and golden brown, about 1 hour.

6. Let the pie rest for 5 minutes before serving. To serve, cut the pie into 4 pieces.

Ingredient tip: This recipe calls for just under 2 cups of beans. If using beans prepared from scratch, soak just under 1 cup of beans to make just under 2 cups cooked beans. This dish works with pinto, Romano, or navy beans. Black or kidney beans will also work in a pinch.

PER SERVING: Calories: 635; Total fat: 29g; Total carbohydrates: 83g; Fiber: 11g; Protein: 14g; Sodium: 935mg

Lentil-Crust Flatbread Pizza

VEGETARIAN, VEGAN (OPTION), GLUTEN-FREE, MAKE AHEAD

SERVES 4 / PREP TIME: 15 MINUTES / COOK TIME: 15 MINUTES (PLUS SOAKING OVERNIGHT)

Lentils are incredibly versatile. Here, they make a delicious flatbread that we're using as a thin-crust–style pizza. Lentils contain protein, iron, and fiber, so they're a nutrient-packed and gluten-free alternative to traditional pizza dough. Top this pizza with any of your favorite pizza toppings. Use canned tomatoes without any added sugar in the ingredients list. This is a fun recipe for a Friday or Saturday night.

FOR THE CRUST

2 cups red lentils

4½ cups water, divided

1 garlic clove

1 tablespoon dried basil

1 tablespoon dried oregano

½ teaspoon salt

½ teaspoon baking powder

1 tablespoon extra-virgin olive oil

FOR THE TOPPINGS

1 cup tomato sauce

½ red bell pepper, sliced

½ green bell pepper, sliced

4 mushrooms, sliced

¼ red onion, thinly sliced

½ cup shredded part-skim mozzarella cheese (or vegan cheese, if desired)

1. Combine the lentils and 4 cups of water in a medium bowl. Soak overnight.
2. Preheat the oven to 400°F.
3. Rinse and drain the lentils and transfer to a food processor.
4. Add the garlic, basil, oregano, salt, baking powder, and remaining ½ cup of water. Purée until smooth.
5. Heat the oil in a skillet over medium heat. Pour in the lentil batter. Smooth the batter out with a spatula, so that it looks like a thin pancake. Make sure the batter is thin. Or divide the batter and fry separately to make individual pizzas.
6. Cook 2 or 3 minutes per side. Then, transfer your flatbreads to a sheet pan covered with parchment paper.
7. Top the flatbread with the tomato sauce and vegetables, and sprinkle with the cheese.
8. Bake in the oven for 15 minutes, until the cheese is bubbling and turning brown.
9. Serve immediately.

Serving tip: Instead of making a pizza with your flatbread, brush it with olive oil while still warm, cut into individual pieces, and serve It alongside dips. It's particularly tasty accompanying Baba Ghanoush (page 66), Beet Hummus (page 73), and Carrot Yogurt Dip (page 68).

PER SERVING: Calories: 420; Total fat: 9g; Total carbohydrates: 61g; Fiber: 29g; Protein: 30g; Sodium: 710mg

Risotto with Green Peas and Lemon

VEGETARIAN, GLUTEN-FREE

SERVES 6 / PREP TIME: 5 MINUTES / COOK TIME: 45 MINUTES

Channel your inner chef to measure out and prepare all the ingredients before you turn on the stove. Cooking risotto is quite involved, so you won't be able to multitask once you get started. As anyone who has watched a chef competition TV show knows, you can't rush risotto. Slow, steady cooking and almost constant stirring is necessary for this true comfort food. It doesn't require any advanced cooking skill. It's just a lot of stirring—you can skip your arm workout at the gym. In this way, risotto is a labor of love.

2 cups frozen peas

3 tablespoons butter

1 cup yellow onion, diced (1 onion)

½ teaspoon salt

1 garlic clove, minced

2 cups arborio rice

3 cups vegetable stock

1 cup white wine

2 tablespoons lemon juice

Grated Parmesan cheese, for garnish (optional)

1. Measure out your peas and leave them on the counter to start defrosting while you prepare the other ingredients.

2. Melt the butter in your largest pot over low-medium heat. Add the onion and salt. Sauté, stirring, for 5 minutes. Add the garlic and sauté, stirring, for another 30 seconds.

3. Add the rice. Increase the heat to medium and stir well to coat the rice in the butter, cooking for 1 minute. Add the peas and pour in a small amount of stock to just cover the rice. Stir. As it dries out, pour in a little more stock.

4. Once the stock runs out, add the wine, little by little, in the same manner as you added the stock.

5. Add the lemon juice.

6. If the risotto is not yet cooked, keep adding warm water (or stock or wine), little by little, until it's soft. You will know that the rice is ready when you see the opacity of the rice change.

7. Serve topped with Parmesan cheese, if using.

Ingredient tip: To get the creamiest risotto, warm your stock in a separate small saucepan and use room-temperature wine.

PER SERVING: Calories: 349; Total fat: 6g; Total carbohydrates: 60g; Fiber: 4g; Protein: 7g; Sodium: 457mg

Baked Spaghetti Squash with Tomato–Black Bean Sauce

VEGETARIAN, VEGAN (OPTION), GLUTEN-FREE, MAKE AHEAD (OPTION)

SERVES 4 / PREP TIME: 10 MINUTES / COOK TIME: 1 HOUR AND 10 MINUTES

Spaghetti squash—named because the flesh is naturally stringy, similar to the pasta—takes the place of wheat-based noodles in this easy dish. Don't be intimidated by the cook time; this can actually be a really quick meal. Simply bake the squash the night before and reheat it in the microwave to pair with the sauce. Voilà, you've got dinner in 15 minutes.

2 spaghetti squash

1 tablespoon extra-virgin olive oil

½ cup diced yellow onion (½ onion)

1 garlic clove, minced

2 cups tomato sauce

1 (15½-ounce) can black beans, drained and rinsed

1 tablespoon dried oregano

1 teaspoon dried basil

¼ teaspoon salt

¼ teaspoon ground black pepper

½ cup fresh Italian flat-leaf parsley, chopped

Grated Parmesan cheese, for garnish (optional)

1. Preheat the oven to 400°F.

2. Put the whole squash in a large, metal baking dish. Cover with a piece of foil, shiny side facing down. Roast until the squash is soft to the touch, about 1 hour.

3. Heat the oil in a large skillet over medium heat. Add the onions and sauté, stirring, for 2 minutes. Add the garlic and sauté for 30 seconds. Add the tomato sauce, beans, oregano, basil, salt, and pepper. Sauté, stirring frequently, for 10 minutes. Add the parsley for the final 1 minute of cooking.

4. Cut the squash open horizontally so that you have 4 ovals. Scoop out the seeds. Transfer one oval each to 4 serving dishes. Rake the flesh with a fork to separate the "noodle" strands.

5. Divide the tomato sauce among the 4 squash. Serve sprinkled with Parmesan cheese, if using.

Make ahead tip: Roast the squash on an evening when you have the time. Split the squash open and scoop out the flesh. Store in a resealable storage container in the refrigerator for up to 3 or 4 days.

PER SERVING: Calories: 287; Total fat: 4g; Total carbohydrates: 57g; Fiber: 7g; Protein: 7g; Sodium: 876mg

Acorn Squash with Wild Rice and Cashew Cream

VEGETARIAN, VEGAN, GLUTEN-FREE, MAKE AHEAD

SERVES 4 / PREP TIME: 10 MINUTES / COOK TIME: 45 MINUTES, PLUS TIME FOR SOAKING

This is a perfect dish for date night or a dinner party. It elegantly embodies the flavors of fall. It's vegan and gluten-free, so it fits many diet choices. While the cooking time is long for this dish, there is hardly any prep involved. You can be cleaning your house and setting the table while it cooks. Don't we all do a frantic house clean before guests arrive?

1 cup cashews

6 cups plus 4 tablespoons water, divided

2 acorn squash

2 cups wild rice

¾ teaspoon salt, divided

¼ teaspoon ground black pepper

1. The night before (or in the morning), in a small bowl, combine the cashews and 2 cups of water. Cover and put in the refrigerator.

2. Preheat the oven to 400°F.

3. Cut the stem off the squash. Cut each squash in half lengthwise (from stem end to pointy end). Scoop out the seeds and place, cut-side up, in a baking dish. Add a teaspoon of water to each seed cavity. Cover with foil and bake until soft, about 45 minutes.

4. In a large saucepan, combine the wild rice with 4 cups of water. Cover and bring to a boil over high heat. Then lower the heat to low and simmer until the rice is soft, about 45 minutes.

5. Drain the cashews, reserving ½ cup of the soaking liquid.

6. In a blender, combine the soaked cashews with ½ teaspoon of salt and ¼ cup of the soaking liquid. Purée until smooth. Add more water, 1 tablespoon at a time, until you reach the desired consistency of a thick sauce. Stop the blender to scrape down the sides several times during puréeing.

7. To serve, put one squash half on each plate and stuff with the wild rice. Pour the cashew cream over top. Season with salt and pepper.

Storage tip: Each component of this dish stores well, but the dish doesn't store well when combined. Store the rice, squash, and cashew cream in separate containers in the refrigerator for 3 or 4 days. Combine the ingredients before reheating.

PER SERVING: Calories: 586; Total fat: 13g; Total carbohydrates: 101g; Fiber: 7g; Protein: 18g; Sodium: 532mg

9

SO-EASY SIDES

ROASTED BRUSSELS SPROUTS
WITH PAPRIKA, PAGE 170

Orange, Cucumber, and Jicama Salad

VEGETARIAN, VEGAN, GLUTEN-FREE

SERVES 4 / TOTAL TIME: 15 MINUTES

Once upon a time, I found a salad recipe in a cookbook that called for jicama. I had no idea what it was. I sought it out and tried it, and I absolutely loved it. I couldn't believe what I had been missing all those years! If you've never had jicama, I encourage you to try it in this refreshing salad recipe. It's one of my go-to recipes for summer barbeque potlucks because I want to introduce other people to jicama, too.

FOR THE SALAD

4 oranges

2 cups jicama

2 cups cucumber

1 cup cilantro, finely chopped (optional)

FOR THE DRESSING

4 tablespoons white wine vinegar

1 tablespoon apple cider vinegar

1 tablespoon lime juice

2 tablespoons extra-virgin olive oil

⅛ teaspoon salt

⅛ teaspoon ground black pepper

1. Peel the oranges, jicama, and the cucumber. Cut the jicama and cucumber into bite-size pieces. Section the orange. Combine the oranges, jicama, and cucumber in a serving bowl. Add the cilantro, if using.
2. In a jar with a tight-fitting lid, combine the dressing ingredients. Shake well. Pour over the salad, tossing to combine.

Preparation tip: Taste the dressing before you add it to the salad. Adjust any ingredients to suit your preferences.

PER SERVING: Calories: 161; Total fat: 7g; Total carbohydrates: 23g; Fiber: 7g; Protein: 2g; Sodium: 76mg

Build Your Own Slaw

VEGETARIAN, VEGAN (OPTION), GLUTEN-FREE, MAKES GREAT LEFTOVERS

SERVES 4 / TOTAL TIME: 10 MINUTES

Slaw doesn't get the respect that it deserves. It's a salad that works all year round. Perfect for picnics, it also tastes great with the veggies that are in-season in the winter. This is more of a technique than a recipe. Mix and match your ingredients and your dressings to suit your taste buds and the season. A food processor's shredding blade makes this really fast. If you don't have a food processor, a hand grater works well. Here, I share my favorite creamy dressing. For a vegan option, use vegan mayonnaise or choose an apple cider or balsamic vinaigrette.

FOR THE SALAD

Choose 4 cups of the following vegetables and fruit:

> Green cabbage
>
> Red cabbage
>
> Kohlrabi
>
> Celeriac
>
> Beets
>
> Carrots
>
> Brussels sprouts
>
> Apple
>
> Pear
>
> Asian pear (also known as apple pear)
>
> ¼ cup raisins (optional)

FOR THE DRESSING

3 tablespoons mayonnaise (or vegan mayonnaise)

2 tablespoons apple cider vinegar

¼ teaspoon pepper

⅛ teaspoon salt

1. Shred the vegetables and fruit. Put them in a serving bowl.
2. Combine the mayonnaise, apple cider vinegar, pepper, and salt in a jar with a tight-fitting lid. Cover with the lid and shake to mix.
3. Pour the dressing over the slaw. Toss to mix well.

Ingredient tip: Shred extra veggies or fruit for leftovers. To prevent veggies from drying out, pour a little olive oil in the storage container and toss with the veggies. To prevent shredded apple from turning brown, add a touch of lemon juice or vinegar.

PER SERVING (INCLUDES GREEN CABBAGE, RED CABBAGE, KOHLRABI, AND CELERIAC): Calories: 106; Total fat: 8g; Total carbohydrates: 8g; Fiber: 3g; Protein: 2g; Sodium: 181mg

PER SERVING (DRESSING ONLY): Calories: 67; Total fat: 7g; Total carbohydrates: 0g; Fiber: 0g; Protein: 0g; Sodium: 125mg

Roasted Brussels Sprouts with Paprika

VEGETARIAN, VEGAN, GLUTEN-FREE, MAKES GREAT LEFTOVERS

SERVES 4 / PREP TIME: 5 MINUTES / COOK TIME: 25 MINUTES

Brussels sprouts were the last vegetable I learned to enjoy. Like many people, as a child I was served them boiled to a mushy death. With their resurgence in popularity over the last 10 years, I tried many a dish where their taste was covered up by bacon, butter, and/or booze. After discovering I enjoyed cauliflower when roasted, I applied that same cooking method to Brussels sprouts, and I loved them! Roasting brings out a caramelizing flavor and mellows their sulfuric flavor. The paprika pairs perfectly, complementing (not masking) the sprouts. Give them another chance with this recipe.

2 tablespoons extra-virgin olive oil

4 cups Brussels sprouts

1 teaspoon paprika

¼ teaspoon salt

1. Preheat the oven to 375°F.
2. Add the oil to a metal baking dish or sheet pan.
3. Remove the loose outer leaves and tough stems from the Brussels sprouts. Cut the sprouts in half lengthwise. If you have some larger sprouts, cut them in quarters so all your sprout pieces are about the same size.
4. Add the sprouts, paprika, and salt to the baking dish. Toss the sprouts to coat well in the oil. Then spread the sprouts in an even layer and roast in the oven for 25 minutes, stirring once halfway through.

Ingredient tip: Paprika is made from dried red bell peppers. The paprika found commonly in supermarkets is technically sweet paprika. If you have access to a store that sells specialty spices, try this recipe with smoked (Spanish) paprika, also called pimenton. Or, if you like the heat, try this recipe with hot (Hungarian) paprika.

PER SERVING: Calories: 99; Total fat: 7g; Total carbohydrates: 8g; Fiber: 3g; Protein: 3g; Sodium: 167mg

FILL THAT OVEN

When turning on the oven to cook one meal, fill the oven with ingredients for other meals. For example:

- **Yams and beets.** Leave beets and yams whole, with their skins on. Rub them with a drop of olive oil and wrap inside a piece of foil, shiny side in. Bake yams until they are soft to the touch, 45 minutes to 1 hour, depending on the size of your yam. Bake beets until you can smell the roasted beet aroma, about 1 to 2 hours, depending on the size of your beet. Dice the roasted yams to add to a salad bowl, or reheat them in the microwave for a quick side on a rushed weeknight dinner. Diced beets are delicious in a salad, or use them for Super Easy Beet Salad (page 172), Pink Pickled Eggs (page 34), or Beet Hummus (page 73).

- **Root veggies.** Oven-Roasted Root Vegetable Fries (page 177) is an incredibly adaptable recipe. Reheat your veggies for a side on a busy weeknight, eat them cold as a root vegetable salad, add them to a salad bowl, or pair them with a handful of nuts for an afternoon snack.

- **Beyond root veggies.** Now that you know the technique for root veggies, expand your horizons beyond the roots. Fennel, broccoli, Brussels sprouts, and cauliflower all taste great roasted (see Roasted Cauliflower with Cumin and Ginger, page 175). Roast an eggplant for Baba Ghanoush (page 66). Cut a winter squash, such as acorn or butternut, in half, scoop out the seeds, put it in a baking dish, add a dash of water in the cavity, and cover it with foil. Bake until soft, 45 minutes to 1 hour. Reheat for a quick side, or eat it cold in a salad.

Super Easy Beet Salad

VEGETARIAN, GLUTEN-FREE, MAKE AHEAD

SERVES 2 / PREP TIME: 5 MINUTES / COOK TIME: 2 HOURS

This fantastic winter "salad" couldn't be any easier or tastier. This recipe was inspired by a salad I once ate at a French cafe. I'm sure that they made their mayonnaise from scratch. Feel free to do the same, but then this salad wouldn't be "super easy." What makes this salad super easy is that you can cook the beets ahead of time. Simply put the beets in the oven when cooking another dish. Make the dressing immediately before serving and enjoy the salad.

2 medium beets

1 teaspoon extra-virgin olive oil, divided

1 tablespoon mayonnaise

1 teaspoon Dijon mustard

1. Preheat the oven to 375°F.
2. Wash, but don't peel, the beets. Cut off the stem at the top and any roots.
3. Lay two pieces of foil on a flat work surface, shiny side up. Drizzle a little olive oil onto the center of each piece of foil. Roll the beet in the olive oil to coat. Then, wrap the beets tightly in the foil. Transfer to a sheet pan. Roast in the oven 1 or 2 hours, or until the beets are cooked through.
4. Allow the beets to cool. Peel the beets and cut into bite-size pieces.
5. In a serving bowl, mix together the mayonnaise and the mustard.
6. Toss the beets in the dressing.

Preparation tip: Adjust the ratio of mayonnaise and mustard to your liking.

PER SERVING: Calories: 103; Total fat: 7g; Total carbohydrates: 8g; Fiber: 2g; Protein: 1g; Sodium: 159mg

Swiss Chard with Capers and Raisins

VEGETARIAN, VEGAN, GLUTEN-FREE

SERVES 4 / PREP TIME: 5 MINUTES / COOK TIME: 10 MINUTES

Don't let the strange-sounding combination of ingredients keep you away from this recipe. It's got the perfect harmony of sweetness from the raisins, saltiness from the capers, and bitterness from the Swiss chard. This recipe doesn't make good leftovers, so only make as much as you'll eat tonight. If you divide the recipe in half, I recommend keeping the full clove of garlic and reducing the raisins to 2 tablespoons. This is an excellent side for seafood dishes, such as Lemon-Garlic Shrimp Kebabs (page 118) and Salmon with Lentils (page 132).

2 tablespoons extra-virgin olive oil

½ cup yellow onion, diced (½ onion)

1 garlic clove

4 cups Swiss chard, coarsely chopped

¼ cup raisins

2 tablespoons capers

⅛ teaspoon ground black pepper

1. Heat the oil in a large skillet over low-medium heat. Add the onion and sauté, stirring, for 4 minutes, until translucent. Add the garlic and continue to cook, stirring, for 30 seconds. Add the chard, raisins, capers, and pepper. Sauté for 5 minutes, until the chard is wilted.
2. Serve immediately.

Ingredient tip: Spinach and kale also work in this recipe. Reduce the sauté time to 3 minutes for spinach. Increase the sauté time to 8 minutes for kale.

PER SERVING: Calories: 104; Total fat: 7g; Total carbohydrates: 11g; Fiber: 1g; Protein: 1g; Sodium: 206mg

Red Cabbage with Apples and Cloves

VEGETARIAN, VEGAN, GLUTEN-FREE

SERVES 4 / PREP TIME: 5 MINUTES / COOK TIME: 40 MINUTES

This sweet-tasting cabbage dish tastes more like dessert than a side dish. You really do want to use red cabbage for this recipe—green cabbage just doesn't pair as well with the apples and spices. Take your time to cook the onions slowly to bring out their natural sweetness. This recipe goes particularly well with pork, such as Pork Tenderloin with White Wine Sauce (page 101).

1 tablespoon extra-virgin olive oil

1 cup yellow onion, diced (1 onion)

4 cups red cabbage, sliced

2 apples, peeled and chopped

¼ teaspoon cloves

1 teaspoon cinnamon

2 tablespoons apple cider vinegar

⅛ teaspoon salt

1. In a large pot, heat the oil over low-medium heat. Add the onion and sauté, stirring, for 4 minutes, until translucent.
2. Increase the heat to medium and add the cabbage and apples. Mix well. Then add the remaining ingredients.
3. Cover the pan and simmer for 35 minutes, until the cabbage is soft.

PER SERVING: Calories: 105; Total fat: 4g; Total carbohydrates: 20g; Fiber: 4g; Protein: 2g; Sodium: 98mg

Roasted Cauliflower with Cumin and Ginger

VEGETARIAN, VEGAN, GLUTEN-FREE

SERVES 2 / PREP TIME: 5 MINUTES / COOK TIME: 20 MINUTES

I admit that I've never been much of a cauliflower fan. Yes, I'd eat it if it was put in front of me, but I never chose it. Now that I have discovered this recipe, I make it every week all winter long! When roasting the cauliflower, look for it to have a lot of dark-brown spots (but not burnt). This will create a sweet, roasted flavor. If you take it out too early, it will be pale, limp, and flavorless. Note that this dish doesn't taste nearly as good as leftovers, so only make as much cauliflower as you think you'll eat tonight.

4 cups cauliflower

2-by-1-inch piece ginger, minced

2 tablespoons olive oil

1 teaspoon cumin

1. Preheat the oven to 425°F.
2. Chop the cauliflower into ¼-inch slices.
3. On a sheet pan, combine all of the ingredients, tossing to combine well.
4. Roast for 20 minutes. Stir the cauliflower twice during cooking.

Ingredient tip: This is a very flexible recipe. Love ginger? Add more. Find the cumin too strong? Use less.

PER SERVING: Calories: 172; Total fat: 14g; Total carbohydrates: 11g; Fiber: 5g; Protein: 4g; Sodium: 60mg

Parsnips with Apples and Oranges

VEGETARIAN, GLUTEN-FREE

SERVES 2 / PREP TIME: 10 MINUTES / COOK TIME: 40 MINUTES

I'm sharing another recipe for parsnips, because they don't get the attention they deserve. This sweet fall and winter recipe will make a veggie lover out of most people! I often recommend this recipe for parents who complain that their picky eater kids won't eat vegetables. This recipe doesn't make great leftovers, so make only enough parsnips to eat for dinner tonight. The recipe is easily divided in half using 3 tablespoons of butter.

2 cups parsnips

2 apples

2 oranges

1 teaspoon orange zest (from 1 orange)

5 tablespoons butter, melted

Dash nutmeg

1. Preheat the oven to 350°F.
2. Peel the parsnips and cut into sticks (similar to how you would prepare carrot sticks). Dice the apples. Peel and slice the oranges.
3. Put the parsnips and fruit into a large bowl.
4. Mix the orange zest, butter, and nutmeg in the baking dish. Stir to combine.
5. Add the parsnips, apples, and oranges and toss to coat.
6. Cover with foil and bake for 30 minutes.
7. Uncover and bake for 10 minutes longer.

Ingredient tip: Look for smaller parsnips. When parsnips grow large, their center becomes woody. If you can only find large parsnips, cut out the woody center before cutting into sticks.

PER SERVING: Calories: 522; Total fat: 30g; Total carbohydrates: 67g; Fiber: 13g; Protein: 4g; Sodium: 222mg

Oven-Roasted Root Vegetable Fries

VEGETARIAN, VEGAN, GLUTEN-FREE, MAKES GREAT LEFTOVERS

SERVES 4 / PREP TIME: 10 MINUTES / COOK TIME: 45 MINUTES

Roasted root vegetables are a staple in my house all fall and winter long. I often add a sheet pan of roasted root vegetables to my oven when I am using it for another dish. Roasted root veggies make great leftovers for a warm side dish or enjoy them cold as a root vegetable salad for lunch. I enjoy them as an afternoon snack paired with a handful of almonds. Note that rutabaga goes by many names. You may know it as turnip (the larger variety) or Swede.

2 tablespoons

extra-virgin olive oil

1 cup sweet potatoes,

cut into ½-inch fries

1 cup parsnips, cut

into ½-inch fries

1 cup rutabaga, cut

into ½-inch fries

1 cup beets, cut into ½-inch fries

1 tablespoon rosemary

1 teaspoon salt

1. Preheat the oven to 425°F.
2. Pour the oil onto a sheet pan. Add the vegetables, rosemary, and salt. Toss to coat the vegetables. Spread everything out to create one layer.
3. Roast for 45 minutes, flipping the vegetables and rotating the sheet pan halfway through roasting.

Ingredient tip: Mix and match your root vegetables in this recipe. For example, carrots, potatoes, and celeriac all work well. Play with the seasoning, too. For example, smoked paprika is a tasty alternative to the rosemary.

PER SERVING: Calories: 150; Total fat: 7g; Total carbohydrates: 21g; Fiber: 4g; Protein: 2g; Sodium: 623mg

Hasselback Yams

VEGETARIAN, GLUTEN-FREE

SERVES 4 / PREP TIME: 10 MINUTES / COOK TIME: 1 HOUR

Hasselback potatoes (and yams) are a chef-y way to make baked potatoes. The slices both show off extra knife skills and allow the garlic-buttery goodness to sink deep into the potatoes. Yes, they take extra work, but they really are impressive. Serve this dish when you want to show extra love for a Sunday family meal or to make a good impression at a dinner party.

4 equal-size yams, unpeeled

1 head garlic

¼ cup unsalted butter

½ teaspoon salt

1 tablespoon rosemary

1. Preheat the oven to 425°F.

2. Choose yams that naturally have a flat spot and will sit still. Cut ¼-inch vertical slices into the yams, stopping before you cut all the way through the bottom. Place on a sheet pan.

3. Reserve two cloves of garlic. For the remaining garlic, remove the outer skin (the loose stuff) and break into individual cloves. Sprinkle them around the sheet pan.

4. In a small saucepan, combine the butter, salt, and rosemary. Mince the 2 remaining garlic cloves and add to the butter mixture. Melt the butter over medium heat. Pour half the butter over the yams. Pick up the yams and rub butter onto the bottom of each one.

5. Bake the yams for 60 minutes, pouring the second half of the butter mixture over them at the halfway point.

Ingredient tip: Yams are higher in vitamins and have a lower glycemic index than regular potatoes, making them a more nutritious choice.

PER SERVING: Calories: 273; Total fat: 21g; Total carbohydrates: 21g; Fiber: 1g; Protein: 3g; Sodium: 404mg

Saffron Quinoa

VEGETARIAN, VEGAN, GLUTEN-FREE

SERVES 4 / PREP TIME: 5 MINUTES / COOK TIME: 20 MINUTES

In this recipe, boring old quinoa is elevated with the exotic but subtle flavor of saffron. Pair this recipe with chicken, lemony fish, or vegetarian recipes involving beans or lentils and tomatoes—such as North African Chickpea Stew (page 143) and Eggplant and Chickpea Stew (page 141). This recipe makes great leftovers, so feel free to double it. Store leftovers in the refrigerator for 3 or 4 days or in a resealable container in the freezer.

⅛ teaspoon saffron threads

1 cup boiling water

½ cup diced yellow onion (½ onion)

2 teaspoons extra-virgin olive oil

1 garlic clove, minced

1 cup quinoa

1 cup water

1. In a small bowl, soak the saffron threads in the boiling water.

2. Heat the oil in a medium saucepan over medium heat. Add the onions and sauté, stirring, for 2 minutes. Add the garlic. Sauté, stirring, for 30 more seconds.

3. Add the quinoa, saffron threads along with their water, and 1 cup of water and stir to combine. Cover and increase heat to high until it comes to a boil. Reduce the heat to low and cook for 15 minutes, until the quinoa is cooked and the water has evaporated. Fluff the quinoa with a fork.

Ingredient tip: Saffron is expensive, but a little goes long way. Saffron is the stamens of a flower. The individual stamens are handpicked. Saffron costs so much because the harvesting process is very labor-intensive.

PER SERVING: Calories: 189; Total fat: 5g; Total carbohydrates: 31g; Fiber: 3g; Protein: 6g; Sodium: 11mg

Peruvian Rice

VEGETARIAN, VEGAN, GLUTEN-FREE, MAKES GREAT LEFTOVERS

SERVES 4 / PREP TIME: 5 MINUTES / COOK TIME: 20 MINUTES

This dish is inspired by my Peruvian-Canadian sweetheart, who blends the traditional ingredients to achieve the flavor he craves without leaving any visible onion pieces about which his (picky) kids will complain. White rice is traditionally served with just about every meal in Lima, Peru, and is used in this recipe. You can substitute brown rice and increase the cooking time to 45 to 60 minutes. This recipe is easiest if you have a blender with measurements on the body of the container. Otherwise, use a measuring cup as you transfer it to the saucepan.

3 Roma tomatoes, coarsely chopped

1 red onion, coarsely chopped

2 garlic cloves

1 cup water

¼ teaspoon salt

2 cups parboiled rice

1. In a blender, combine the tomatoes, onion, garlic, water, and salt. Blend until smooth. You may need to add the ingredients in batches, depending on size of your blender.
2. Top up with extra water if the mixture doesn't measure 4 cups.
3. Pour the mixture into a large saucepan. Add the rice. Cover and bring to a boil over high heat. Stir.
4. Reduce the heat to low and cook, covered, for 20 minutes, or until rice is cooked.

Ingredient tip: Parboiled rice, commonly sold as "converted rice," has more vitamins and minerals than regular white rice. And it has a much lower glycemic index.

PER SERVING: Calories: 379; Total fat: 1g; Total carbohydrates: 82g; Fiber: 1g; Protein: 9g; Sodium: 150mg

Barley Tabouli

VEGETARIAN, VEGAN, MAKES GREAT LEFTOVERS

SERVES 4 / PREP TIME: 10 MINUTES / COOK TIME: 40 MINUTES

This recipe includes two ingredients that are often overlooked: barley and parsley. Barley has lots of fiber, specifically the kind that helps to lower cholesterol, so it's a great substitution for the couscous that is traditionally used in tabouli. Another overlooked ingredient, parsley, is more than just a garnish. It counts as a leafy green vegetable. Feel free to adjust the lemon juice, garlic, salt, and pepper to your taste.

1 cup pearl barley

2 cups water

¼ cup lemon juice (from 1 lemon)

2 cups Italian flat-leaf parsley

2 tablespoons

extra-virgin olive oil

1 garlic clove, minced

¼ teaspoon salt

¼ teaspoon ground black pepper

1. Put the barley and water in a large saucepan. Cover and bring to a boil over high heat. When the water comes to a boil, reduce the heat to low. Simmer for 40 minutes.
2. Chop the parsley. Put the lemon juice, olive oil, parsley, garlic, salt, and pepper in a medium bowl.
3. Add the cooked barley to the parsley mixture. Toss to combine.

Preparation tip: This recipe makes great leftovers. Double the recipe and store in the refrigerator for 3 or 4 days.

PER SERVING: Calories: 252; Total fat: 8g; Total carbohydrates: 42g; Fiber: 9g; Protein: 6g; Sodium: 167mg

Spiced Rice and Peas

VEGETARIAN, VEGAN (OPTION), GLUTEN-FREE, MAKES GREAT LEFTOVERS

SERVES 2 / PREP TIME: 10 MINUTES / COOK TIME: 20 MINUTES

I love how the cuisine of South Asia elevates such simple ingredients, in this case rice and frozen peas, into total deliciousness with complex spices. This is a fantastic accompaniment to vegetarian dishes, such as Coconut Red Lentils (page 142), or poultry dishes, such as Lemon-Garlic Roast Chicken (page 91). It's particularly rich with the butter, but you can substitute olive oil to make this a vegan dish.

½ **cup parboiled rice**

2 **cups boiling water**

¼ **teaspoon ground black pepper**

¼ **teaspoon cinnamon**

¼ **teaspoon cloves**

¼ **teaspoon cardamom**

¼ **teaspoon turmeric**

4 **teaspoons unsalted butter**

1 **shallot, finely diced**

1-by-1-inch **piece of**

fresh ginger, minced

2 **garlic cloves, minced**

½ **cup frozen peas**

⅛ **teaspoon salt**

1. Soak the rice in water while preparing the remaining ingredients.

2. Boil the 2 cups of water in a kettle.

3. Combine the pepper, cinnamon, cloves, cardamom, and turmeric in a small bowl. Set aside.

4. Melt the butter in a large saucepan over medium heat. Sauté the shallot, ginger, and garlic, stirring, for 1 minute.

5. Drain the rice. Add the rice, peas, and the spice mixture to the saucepan. Sauté for 1 minute, stirring.

6. Add the boiling water. Cover, lower the heat to low, and cook for 15 minutes, or until the rice is cooked.

Storage tip: This dish makes great leftovers, so feel free to double it. Store in the refrigerator for 3 or 4 days, or in the freezer for 2 or 3 months.

PER SERVING: Calories: 278; Total fat: 8g; Total carbohydrates: 45g; Fiber: 2g; Protein: 6g; Sodium: 189mg

Moroccan-Inspired Quinoa

VEGETARIAN, VEGAN, GLUTEN-FREE

SERVES 4 / PREP TIME: 5 MINUTES / COOK TIME: 30 MINUTES

In this recipe, quick-cooking quinoa replaces the traditional couscous. Couscous is a refined version of wheat. Quinoa is a whole grain. With this substitution, we've increased the nutritional impact of this dish. Also, this recipe includes turmeric, which has been getting a lot of attention lately for its anti-inflammatory properties. With the sweetness from the raisins and apricots, the deliciousness is all you will notice. It pairs well with vegetarian dishes made with tofu or beans and lentils (chickpeas pair particularly well). It also pairs well with chicken.

3 cups water

1 tablespoon extra-virgin olive oil

½ cup diced yellow onion (about half an onion)

2 garlic cloves, minced

1 cup quinoa

1 teaspoon turmeric

½ teaspoon cumin seeds

¼ cup raisins

¼ cup diced apricots

½ cup slivered almonds

¼ teaspoon salt

¼ teaspoon black pepper

1. Preheat the oven to 350°F.
2. Boil the water.
3. Heat the oil in a large skillet over medium heat. Add the onions and sauté, stirring, for 2 minutes. Add the garlic and sauté for 30 seconds. Add the quinoa, turmeric, and cumin seeds and sauté, stirring, for 1 minute.
4. In an ungreased 9-by-9-inch (1-quart) ceramic or glass baking dish, combine the quinoa mixture, raisins, apricots, almonds, salt, and pepper. Pour in the boiling water. Cover with foil and bake for 20 to 25 minutes, or until the quinoa is cooked.

PER SERVING: Calories: 339; Total fat: 13g; Total carbohydrates: 49g; Fiber: 6g; Protein: 10g; Sodium: 150mg

10

NATURALLY SWEET ENDINGS

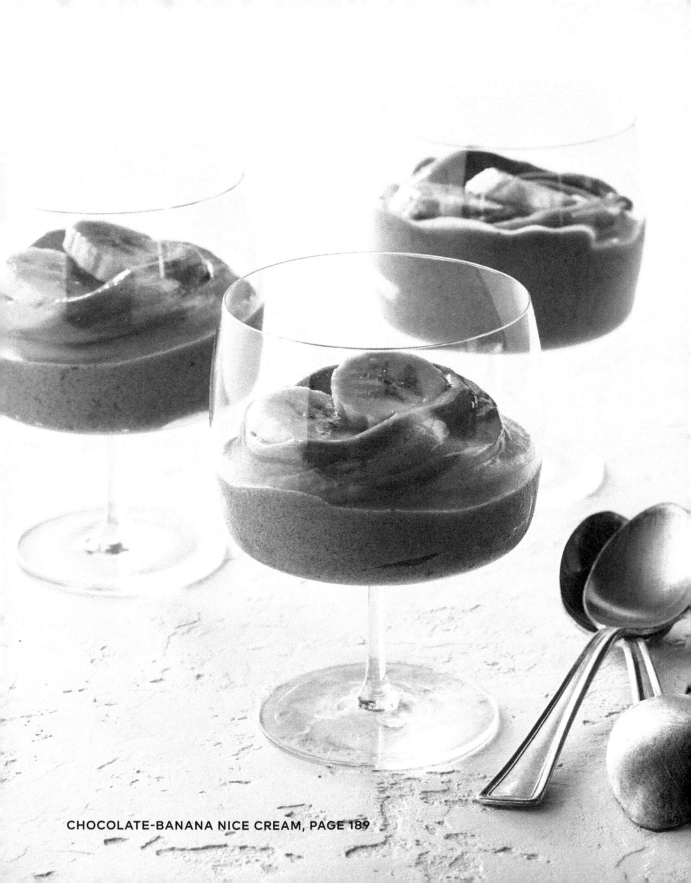

CHOCOLATE-BANANA NICE CREAM, PAGE 189

Fruit Salad with Ginger-Orange-Lime Dressing

VEGETARIAN, VEGAN, GLUTEN-FREE

SERVES 4 / TOTAL TIME: 10 MINUTES

This bright, refreshing dressing turns a simple fruit salad into a dish worthy of being called dessert. It is at home as a way to finish a meal in both summer and winter. This dessert is the perfect end to a light meal on a hot summer evening. It's also a palate-cleansing end to a heavy winter meal. I've also served this as the end of a Sunday brunch.

FOR THE DRESSING

1 tablespoon orange zest (from 1 orange)

½ teaspoon lime zest (from 1 lime)

¼ cup fresh lime juice (3 or 4 limes)

1-by-1-inch piece of ginger, minced

FOR THE SALAD

1 cup diced cantaloupe melon

1 cup diced honeydew melon

1 cup diced watermelon

1 cup diced mango

1. Combine the dressing ingredients in a jar with a tight-fitting lid. Cover and shake to combine.
2. Drizzle the fruit with the dressing and toss to coat.

Ingredient tip: Papaya would be amazing in this fruit salad as well.

PER SERVING: Calories: 71; Total fat: 0g; Total carbohydrates: 18g; Fiber: 2g; Protein: 1g; Sodium: 13mg

OTHER WAYS TO END THE MEAL

Often, we crave food because our bodies have learned an association between a particular food and a particular situation. This is what happens with dessert. If you have always had something sweet at the end of a meal, you are going to crave something sweet when you finish dinner. You will have this craving even if you have eaten enough to be full.

The way to combat this cause of cravings is to establish a new habit or routine. Once this new routine truly becomes a new habit, you won't crave a sugary dessert. Here are some other ways to end a meal. Which one will become your new habit?

- **Choose fresh fruit.** Why not use dessert as an opportunity to get in one more serving of fruit?

- **Choose cheese.** Take inspiration from the French. Finish your meal with some cheese.

- **Choose herbs and spices.** Finish your meal with herbs and spices that have traditionally been used to aid in digestion, such as fennel seeds, or used to freshen breath, such as fresh parsley.

- **Choose tea.** Finish your meal with a cup of herbal tea (without added sugar or honey). Some varieties have sweet flavors without any free sugar, such as apple-cinnamon or mint-chocolate.

Cantaloupe Granita

VEGETARIAN, VEGAN, GLUTEN-FREE, MAKE AHEAD

SERVES 4 / PREP TIME: 10 MINUTES / FREEZING TIME: 4 HOURS

Similar to a slushy but made with real fruit, granitas are refreshing in the summer heat. They're also incredibly easy to prepare. The only trick is to plan ahead, so that you are home and remember to break up the ice crystals every hour. I set the alarm on my phone to remind me. Once you have the technique down, mix and match the fruit in your granita.

4 cups diced cantaloupe

¼ cup fresh lemon juice (juice from 1 lemon)

¼ cup water

1. In a blender, combine the cantaloupe, lemon juice, and water. Purée until the mixture is smooth.
2. Pour into a nonmetal baking dish, such as a reusable plastic container.
3. Put in the freezer. Freeze for 1 hour.
4. Remove from the freezer and scrape thoroughly with a fork, breaking up the ice crystals.
5. Return to the freezer for 1 hour. Again, remove from the freezer and break up the ice crystals with a fork. Repeat at least 2 more times.

Equipment tip: A shallow container works best so that you can easily rake your fork through the mixture to break up the ice crystals.

PER SERVING: Calories: 58; Total fat: 0g; Total carbohydrates: 14g; Fiber: 1g; Protein: 1g; Sodium: 14mg

Chocolate-Banana Nice Cream

VEGETARIAN, VEGAN, GLUTEN-FREE, MAKE AHEAD

SERVES 1 / TOTAL TIME: 5 MINUTES, PLUS OVERNIGHT TO FREEZE

This recipe is creamy, smooth, and delicious—just like ice cream! The best thing about this recipe (besides the taste) is that it only includes two ingredients. Blending the banana does take a little while. At first the slices will break into a chunky slurry, and you will likely think that this "nice cream" idea doesn't work. Be patient. Next it will form one big ball. Then, suddenly, it will become a beautiful, smooth, whipped texture—just like ice cream. There are likely hundreds of flavor combinations. I'm sharing the chocolate version. Try it plain with just the banana or add ¼ teaspoon cinnamon for a delicious combination.

1 cup bananas, peeled and sliced

1 teaspoon cocoa

1. Freeze the bananas overnight.
2. Put frozen sliced bananas and cocoa powder in a blender. Blend until smooth.

Ingredient tip: The secret to this recipe is very ripe bananas. Buy them when you see them in the store, slice, and freeze them. Then you're ready to make nice cream anytime you wish.

PER SERVING: Calories: 138; Total fat: 1g; Total carbohydrates: 35g; Fiber: 4g; Protein: 2g; Sodium: 2mg

Coffee Whipped Cream

VEGETARIAN, GLUTEN-FREE

SERVES 2 / TOTAL TIME: 5 MINUTES

This whipped cream is brilliantly easy. The ½ teaspoon instant coffee indicated creates a whipped cream with just a hint of coffee. Are you a coffee lover? Increase the coffee to 1 teaspoon for an intense coffee flavor. Serve it on its own as a light way to end a summer meal, try it with fresh fruit, or combine it with other recipes in this cookbook—such as Coconut Custard Pie (page 196), White Wine–Poached Pears (page 194), or Chocolate-Avocado-Coconut Pot de Crème (page 192).

1 cup whipping cream

¼ teaspoon cinnamon

¼ teaspoon vanilla extract

½ teaspoon instant

coffee granules

Combine all of the ingredients in an immersion blender or a bowl. Whip the cream with the immersion blender or an egg beater until it forms stiff peaks.

Equipment tip: To get the stiffest peaks, put your bowl and beater in the refrigerator for 30 minutes before you make the whipped cream.

PER SERVING: Calories: 413; Total fat: 44g; Total carbohydrates: 4g; Fiber: 0g; Protein: 2g; Sodium: 45mg

Pumpkin Cheesecake Mousse

VEGETARIAN, GLUTEN-FREE

SERVES 2 / TOTAL TIME: 15 MINUTES

There's no need to miss out on pumpkin spice season just because you're not eating free sugar. This dessert is part cheesecake, part mousse, and all pumpkin spice. Good things come in small packages. This dessert is incredibly rich, so the small serving totally satisfies. An immersion blender is the perfect tool to make this recipe—just wash it between making the mousse and the whipped cream topping. If using a traditional blender for the mousse, pulse it at the beginning to get the ingredients combined. Stop the blender occasionally to scrape down the sides.

⅓ cup cream cheese

⅓ cup canned pumpkin

¼ cup plus 2 tablespoons whipping cream, divided

¼ teaspoon pumpkin pie spice

1. Combine the cream cheese, pumpkin, 2 tablespoons whipping cream, and spices in a blender. Purée the mixture until smooth and airy.
2. Transfer the mixture to two small serving bowls, ramekins, or glasses. Cover and put in the refrigerator.
3. Whip the remaining whipping cream until it forms stiff peaks. Top the two bowls of mousse with the whipped cream.

Ingredient tip: Be sure that you are buying canned pumpkin, not pumpkin pie filling. Pumpkin pie filling contains free sugar. If you cannot find pumpkin pie spice, it can be recreated with ¼ teaspoon cinnamon and a dash of both ground ginger and ground nutmeg.

PER SERVING: Calories: 299; Total fat: 30g; Total carbohydrates: 6g; Fiber: 2g; Protein: 4g; Sodium: 132mg

Chocolate-Avocado-Coconut Pot de Crème

VEGETARIAN, VEGAN, GLUTEN-FREE, MAKE AHEAD

SERVES 2 / TOTAL TIME: 5 MINUTES, PLUS 3 HOURS REFRIGERATION

This recipe is for my fellow dark chocolate lovers. It creates a dense, dark chocolate pudding. An immersion blender works best for this recipe, but it can also be made in a regular blender. Just stop several times during the blending to scrape down the sides. It's extra amazing when topped with whipped cream. Choose plain whipped cream or top it with the Coffee Whipped Cream (page 190).

¼ cup coconut cream (from a can of coconut milk)

2 avocados

¼ cup cocoa powder

1½ teaspoons vanilla extract

1. Put the can of coconut milk in the fridge.
2. In a blender, combine the avocados, cocoa powder, and vanilla.
3. Take the coconut milk out of the refrigerator. Open the can. Scoop off the solid cream that has formed at the top of the can. Add the coconut cream to the blender. Blend until the mixture is smooth.
4. Transfer to two serving glasses or bowls. Cover and refrigerate for 3 hours.

Ingredient tip: I always put two cans of coconut milk in the fridge because you never know how much coconut cream you'll get in a can. If you don't get ¼ cup from one can, you will need two cans of coconut milk.

PER SERVING: Calories: 382; Total fat: 28g; Total carbohydrates: 30g; Fiber: 15g; Protein: 5g; Sodium: 36mg

Strawberries and Goat Cheese Dessert Panini

VEGETARIAN, GLUTEN-FREE (OPTION)

SERVES 2 / PREP TIME: 5 MINTES / COOK TIME: 5 MINUTES

The best way to describe this recipe is to imagine that a grilled cheese sandwich and a dessert had a baby. If you can make a grilled cheese sandwich, you can make this dessert. Here, I share the strange but delicious combination of strawberries, balsamic vinegar, goat cheese, and black pepper (trust me, give it a try). As the seasons change, use different fillings. For example, pair sliced plums or peaches with goat cheese. Or, along with the goat cheese, add sliced pears and a dash of cinnamon. Or, pair sliced apples with Brie.

4 to 6 strawberries

¼ teaspoon balsamic vinegar

Butter

4 pieces whole grain bread (gluten-free, if desired)

3 ounces goat cheese

Dash black pepper

1. Preheat a panini press.
2. Slice the strawberries and put them in a small bowl along with the balsamic vinegar. Toss the strawberries gently to coat in the vinegar.
3. Butter one side of each slice of bread. On the unbuttered side, spread the goat cheese. Top with an even layer of the sliced strawberries. Sprinkle with a dash of black pepper.
4. Close the sandwich.
5. Place in the panini press. Cook until the light indicates that it's done, or the sandwich is golden brown.

Equipment tip: This recipe can be made without a panini press. Put the sandwich in a skillet on low-medium heat and put a pot or other heatproof item on top of the sandwich to weigh it down. Flip the sandwich when it turns golden brown.

PER SERVING: Calories: 386; Total fat: 16g; Total carbohydrates: 48g; Fiber: 11g; Protein: 21g; Sodium: 559mg

White Wine–Poached Pears

VEGETARIAN, VEGAN, GLUTEN-FREE

SERVES 4 / PREP TIME: 5 MINUTES / COOK TIME: 30 MINUTES, PLUS 6 HOURS REFRIGERATION

This recipe is a true celebration of fruit's deliciousness. An elegant dish, it's perfect for a dinner party, and it's so tasty that your guests will never miss the free sugar. While I love eating this dish warm, it can also be made ahead of time (perfect for entertaining) and served chilled. Because the pears are the focus of this recipe, choose firm, ripe pears when they are in season. Thankfully, pears have a long season, from summer right through fall to winter.

1 bottle (750 ml) lighter, fruitier white wine, like Pinot Grigio

¼ cup fresh lemon juice (from 1 lemon)

¼ teaspoon vanilla extract

¼ teaspoon cinnamon

Zest from 1 lemon

4 firm, ripe pears

1. In a large saucepan, combine the wine, lemon juice, vanilla, cinnamon, and lemon zest. Over high heat, cover and bring the mixture to a boil. Remove the lid and cook for 3 minutes. Add the pears, lower the heat to medium, and cook for 20 minutes, until the pears are tender. Halfway through the cooking time, rotate the pears very gently. Remove the pears and set aside. Cover the poaching liquid, increase the heat to high, and bring it to a boil. Remove the cover and allow the liquid to reduce by half, about 5 minutes.

2. Pour the sauce over the pears. Serve the dish immediately or refrigerate, covered, at least 6 hours and serve cold.

Serving tip: This recipe tastes amazing when topped with Coffee Whipped Cream (page 190).

PER SERVING: Calories: 212; Total fat: 0g; Total carbohydrates: 24g; Fiber: 4g; Protein: 1g; Sodium: 13mg

CUT IT OUT (BAKING WITHOUT SUGAR)

Sugar has multiple functions in baking. Whether you can make your recipe without free sugar depends on the function that sugar is performing in the recipe.

Sugar's functions:

- **Structure:** Sugar makes egg whites stiffen for meringues.
- **Moistens:** Sugar is responsible for moistness in many recipes, and it helps create tender baked goods.
- **Browning:** Sugar is responsible for the golden color of cookies, cakes, etc.
- **Sweetness:** Of course, sugar also provides the sweet flavor in baking.

You can replace free sugar with substitutes when it's performing the sweetness and moisture functions. For example, check out the recipes in this chapter, as well as Apple-Cinnamon Muffins (page 79) and Fruit and Nut Squares (page 80) in the Snacks chapter. The color of baking will be different when replacing free sugar in recipes in which it's performing its browning function, but the recipes can still taste delicious. I don't know of any substitutes for free sugar in recipes in which it's performing its structure role with egg whites.

Experiment substituting free sugar with ingredients such as:

- **Fruit purées,** such as applesauce
- **Dried fruit,** such as dates, raisins, and shredded coconut
- **Canned pumpkin**
- **Grated vegetables,** such as zucchini, beets, and carrots
- **Dairy products,** such as ricotta and cream cheese

Coconut Custard Pie

VEGETARIAN

SERVES 8 / PREP TIME: 5 MINUTES / BAKE TIME: 1 HOUR

My friend Debbie introduced me to this recipe. It's the easiest baking recipe I've ever come across. Amazingly, the pie forms two textures while it bakes—an internal custard and an outer crust. One of the classes I took to become a dietitian was called food science. Making pie pastry in this class was the only assignment I ever failed in my eight years of university. To this day, I avoid making pastry at all costs. So, you can understand my excitement when Debbie showed me this recipe where the pie makes its own crust.

Cooking oil spray

½ cup plus ½ tablespoon all-purpose flour, divided

4 large eggs

6 tablespoons butter

2 cups milk

1 teaspoon vanilla extract

1 cup unsweetened, shredded coconut

1. Preheat the oven to 350°F.
2. Coat a 9½-inch glass pie plate with cooking oil spray and dust it with ½ tablespoon of flour.
3. In a blender, combine the eggs, butter, ½ cup of the flour, milk, vanilla, and coconut. Blend until smooth.
4. Pour the batter into the prepared pie plate.
5. Bake for 50 to 60 minutes, until the custard is set and golden brown.

Serving tip: This recipe pairs beautifully with fresh fruit, such as berries.

PER SERVING: Calories: 231; Total fat: 18g; Total carbohydrates: 11g; Fiber: 2g; Protein: 7g; Sodium: 130mg

Free-Form Apple Crumble

VEGETARIAN, GLUTEN-FREE (OPTION), MAKES GREAT LEFTOVERS

SERVES 4 / PREP TIME: 5 MINUTES / BAKE TIME: 30 MINUTES

You can't go wrong with apples, cinnamon, and butter. I don't understand all the fuss with making fancy crumbles. This one has less hassle and all the delicious flavor. Choose a juicy apple variety for this recipe, such as McIntosh. You can also use in-season plums, peaches, and nectarines, just omit the cinnamon. Serve your apple crumble as-is or top it with whipped cream.

4 apples, cored and diced

¼ cup water (if using a drier variety of apple, such as Ambrosia)

½ teaspoon cinnamon

1 cup rolled oats (gluten-free if desired)

¼ cup unsalted butter, cut into small pieces

1. Preheat the oven to 375°F.
2. In a 9-by-13-inch ceramic or glass lasagna pan, spread the apples in one layer. Pour in the water (if using). Sprinkle cinnamon over top of the apples. Top with the oats. Then, distribute the small pieces of butter over top.
3. Bake for 20 to 30 minutes, or until the apples are fragrant and soft. Cooking time will vary with the variety of apple.

Preparation tip: Keep the skins on the apples for extra fiber.

PER SERVING: Calories: 272; Total fat: 13g; Total carbohydrates: 39g; Fiber: 7g; Protein: 3g; Sodium: 4mg

MEASUREMENT CONVERSIONS

VOLUME EQUIVALENTS (LIQUID)

US STANDARD	US STANDARD (OUNCES)	METRIC (APPROXIMATE)
2 tablespoons	1 fl. oz.	30 mL
¼ cup	2 fl. oz.	60 mL
½ cup	4 fl. oz.	120 mL
1 cup	8 fl. oz.	240 mL
1½ cups	12 fl. oz.	355 mL
2 cups or 1 pint	16 fl. oz.	475 mL
4 cups or 1 quart	32 fl. oz.	1 L
1 gallon	128 fl. oz.	4 L

OVEN TEMPERATURES

FAHRENHEIT	CELSIUS (APPROXIMATE)
250°F	120°C
300°F	150°C
325°F	165°C
350°F	180°C
375°F	190°C
400°F	200°C
425°F	220°C
450°F	230°C

VOLUME EQUIVALENTS (DRY)

US STANDARD	METRIC (APPROXIMATE)
⅛ teaspoon	0.5 mL
¼ teaspoon	1 mL
½ teaspoon	2 mL
¾ teaspoon	4 mL
1 teaspoon	5 mL
1 tablespoon	15 mL
¼ cup	59 mL
⅓ cup	79 mL
½ cup	118 mL
⅔ cup	156 mL
¾ cup	177 mL
1 cup	235 mL
2 cups or 1 pint	475 mL
3 cups	700 mL
4 cups or 1 quart	1 L

WEIGHT EQUIVALENTS

US STANDARD	METRIC (APPROXIMATE)
½ ounce	15 g
1 ounce	30 g
2 ounces	60 g
4 ounces	115 g
8 ounces	225 g
12 ounces	340 g
16 ounces or 1 pound	455 g

THE DIRTY DOZEN AND THE CLEAN FIFTEEN™

A nonprofit environmental watchdog organization called Environmental Working Group (EWG) looks at data supplied by the US Department of Agriculture (USDA) and the Food and Drug Administration (FDA) about pesticide residues. Each year it compiles a list of the best and worst pesticide loads found in commercial crops. You can use these lists to decide which fruits and vegetables to buy organic to minimize your exposure to pesticides and which produce is considered safe enough to buy conventionally. This does not mean they are pesticide-free, though, so wash these fruits and vegetables thoroughly. The list is updated annually, and you can find it online at EWG.org/FoodNews.

Dirty Dozen™

1. strawberries
2. spinach
3. kale
4. nectarines
5. apples
6. grapes
7. peaches
8. cherries
9. pears
10. tomatoes
11. celery
12. potatoes

† *Additionally, nearly three-quarters of hot pepper samples contained pesticide residues.*

Clean Fifteen™

1. avocados
2. sweet corn*
3. pineapples
4. sweet peas (frozen)
5. onions
6. papayas*
7. eggplants
8. asparagus
9. kiwis
10. cabbages
11. cauliflower
12. cantaloupes
13. broccoli
14. mushrooms
15. honeydew melons

* *A small amount of sweet corn, papaya, and summer squash sold in the United States is produced from genetically modified seeds. Buy organic varieties of these crops if you want to avoid genetically modified produce.*

REFERENCES

Chapter 1

WHAT IS SUGAR?

Canadian Sugar Institute. http://sugar.ca Accessed May 17, 2019.

Sugar Science: The Unsweetened Truth. University of California San Francisco. http://sugarscience.ucsf.edu/hidden-in-plain-sight/#.XSJ3zJNKgWp . Accessed May 17, 2019.

World Health Organization. 2015. Guideline: Sugars Intake for Adults and Children. https://www.who.int/nutrition/publications/guidelines/sugars_intake/en/. Accessed May 17, 2019.

FRUCTOSE'S BAD RAP

Sun, S.Z. & Empie, M.W. 2012. Fructose metabolism in humans—what isotopic tracer studies tell us. *Nutrition & Metabolism*, 9, 89. doi.org/10.1186/1743-7075-9-89.

Khan, T.A. & Sievenpiper, J.L. 2016. Controversies about sugars: results from systematic reviews and meta-analyses on obesity, cardiometabolic disease and diabetes. *Eur J Nutr* 55(Suppl 2): 25. doi.org/10.1007/s00394-016-1345-3.

Evans, G.H., McLaughlin, J.M., Yau, A.M.W. 2018. The effect of glucose or fructose added to a semi-solid meal on gastric emptying rate, appetite, and blood chemistry. *Frontiers in Nutrition*. 5:94. doi.org/10.3389/fnut.2018.00094.

WHAT HAPPENS WHEN YOU EAT SUGAR?

Rada, P., Avena, N.M., Hoelel, B.G. 2005. Daily bingeing on sugar repeatedly releases dopamine in the accumbens shell. *Neuroscience*. 134(3). doi.org/10.1016/j.neuroscience.2005.04.043.

Mergenthaler, P., Lindauer, U., Dienel, G.A., & Meisel, A. 2013. Sugar for the brain: the role of glucose in physiological and pathological brain function. *Trends in Neuroscience* 36(10) 587-597. doi.org/10.1016/j.tins.2013.07.001.

IS IT POSSIBLE TO BE ADDICTED TO SUGAR

Canadian Mental Health Association. http://ontario.cmha.ca/addiction-and-substance-use-and-addiction/ Accessed May 17, 2019.

American Psychiatric Association. 2013. *Diagnostic and Statistical Manual of Mental Disorders* (DSM-5), Fifth Edition.

Westwater, M.L., Fletcher, P.C. & Ziauddeen, H. 2016. Sugar addiction: the state of the science. *Eur J Nutr* 55(Suppl 2): 55. doi.org/10.1007/s00394-016-1229-6.

Chapter 2

YOU CALL IT MALTITOL, I CALL IT SUGAR
Sugar Science: The Unsweetened Truth. University of California San Francisco. http://sugarscience.ucsf.edu/hidden-in-plain-sight/#.XSJ3zJNKgWp. Accessed May 17, 2019.

Chapter 6

HOW LONG DO THOSE LEFTOVERS KEEP?
US Food and Drug Administration. Are you Storing Food Safely? https://www.fda.gov/consumers/consumer-updates/are-you-storing-food-safely. Accessed August 21, 2019.

US Food and Drug Administration. Refrigerator and Freezer Storage Chart. https://www.fda.gov/media/74435/download. Accessed June 9, 2019.

Government of Canada. Safe Food Storage. https://www.canada.ca/en/health-canada/services/general-food-safety-tips/safe-food-storage.html. Accessed August 21, 2019.

Fight Bac! www.fightbac.org. Accessed June 9, 2019.

Chapter 7

HOW TO SAFELY THAW FROZEN FISH
US Food and Drug Administration. Fresh and Frozen Seafood. https://www.fda.gov/media/79895/download. Accessed August 21, 2019.

INDEX

ABOUT THE AUTHOR

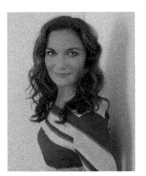

Kristen Yarker, MSc, RD, is a registered dietitian-nutritionist and lives in Victoria, British Columbia, Canada. With 24 years of nutrition experience, Kristen creates practical, custom solutions for busy people to successfully adopt healthy eating habits for both performance and pleasure. Kristen is a sought-after speaker, writer, and consultant to health organizations. When not working, you'll find Kristen shopping at farmers' markets, trail running, surfing, and practicing yoga.